Quick G

Quick Guide to Hematology Testing

Vishnu Reddy, MD
Professor, Department of Pathology
Division of Laboratory Medicine and Anatomic Pathology
Hematopathology Director
The University of Alabama at Birmingham
Birmingham, Alabama

Marisa B. Marques, MD
Associate Professor, Department of Pathology
Division of Laboratory Medicine
Transfusion Medicine and Coagulation Service Director
The University of Alabama at Birmingham
Birmingham, Alabama

George A. Fritsma, MS, MT(ASCP)
Associate Professor, Pathology and Clinical Laboratory Science
University of Alabama at Birmingham
Birmingham, Alabama

AACCPress

1850 K Street, NW, Suite 625
Washington, DC 20006

1 2 3 4 5 6 7 8 9 0   EB 09 08 07

Printed in the United States of America

Library of Congress Cataloging-in-Publication Data

Reddy, Vishnu
    Quick guide to hematology testing / Vishnu Reddy, Marisa B. Marques, George A. Fritsma.
       p. ; cm.
    Includes bibliographical references.
    ISBN 978-1-59425-074-3

    1. Blood—Examination—Handbooks, manuals, etc. 2. Diagnosis, Laboratory—Handbooks, manuals, etc. 3. Hematology—Handbooks, manuals, etc. I. Marques, Marisa B. II. Fritsma, George A. III. American Association for Clinical Chemistry. IV. Title.
    [DNLM: 1. Hematologic Tests—methods—Handbooks. QY 39 R313q 2007]

    RB45.R34 2007
    616.07'561—dc22

                                                                2007009095

Contents

Hematology Specimens

Collecting Anticoagulated Whole Blood for Complete Blood Counts (CBCs)

1. Establish the identity of the patient (1).
2. Collect blood into a lavender-topped evacuated tube coated with dipotassium ethylene diamine tetraacetic acid (K_2EDTA). Fill to the *proper level* determined by internal pressure reduction. Short draws result in *distorted cellular morphology* and should be avoided.
3. Gently invert 8–10 times to mix.
4. In the presence of the patient, label the tube with the *patient's full name, medical record number, date and time of collection, and phlebotomist identification*.
5. Transport to the laboratory upright within *one hour of collection* at room temperature.

Collecting Capillary Whole Blood for CBCs

1. Puncture the skin to provide free-flowing capillary blood; discard the first drop (2).
2. Prepare blood films before filling the micro specimen container.
3. Collect the specimen in an EDTA-coated micro specimen container, filling to the proper level.
4. Gently invert 8–10 times to mix.
5. In the presence of the patient, attach a label with the *patient's full name, medical record number, date and time of collection and phlebotomist identification*.
6. Transport to the laboratory upright within *one hour of collection* at room temperature.

Specimen Collection Requirements and Errors

- *Mixing:* The specimen partially clots if not inverted 8–10 times immediately after collection. Even a small clot profoundly changes test results and necessitates a re-draw (3).

- *Shaking:* The specimen should never be shaken. Shaking ruptures red blood cells (RBCs), causing hemolysis with erroneous RBC counts, hematocrit (HCT) results, and RBC indices.

- *Short draw:* Evacuated tubes are designed to collect specific volumes ranging from 2.0 to 10.0 mL. The hematopathology laboratory director selects the preferred tube volumes. Phlebotomists allow each tube to fill completely, as controlled by internal pressure reduction. The proper concentration is 1.5 mg K_2EDTA per mL blood. A "short draw" causes an increased anticoagulant-to-blood ratio and shrinks blood cells, causing morphologic distortion, inaccurate RBC count, and HCT results, and altered blood film staining.

- *Capillary specimens* collected in EDTA are necessary when testing infants and adults for whom venipuncture is contraindicated by poor veins or risk of multiple collections.

Specimen Management Requirements

- The specimen is stored at room temperature; 18 °C to 24 °C Specimens are only stored at refrigerator temperature, 2 °C to 8 °C, for protocols established by the laboratory director.

- Blood films are prepared within two hours of collection to avoid white blood cell (WBC), RBC, and platelet distortion.

- A valid CBC may be produced up to 24 hours after collection; however specimen storage limits are set by individual laboratory personnel and vary by analyzer technology.

- Blood from capillary punctures must be analyzed within four hours of collection.

- Specimens must be inverted 8–10 times just prior to testing.

- Capillary specimens must be inverted 20 times just prior to testing.

Spurious Thrombocytopenia

In 0.2% of patients, K_2EDTA exposes a platelet antigen that binds a natural antibody (4). Platelets adhere to polymorphonuclear neutrophils (PMNs) and sometimes monocytes (MONOs), easily visualized on the blood film as "*platelet satellitosis.*" Satellitosis produces a false, *markedly reduced platelet count.* Spurious thrombocytopenia is a laboratory nuisance with no clinical significance. A new specimen should be collected using a blue-topped 3.2% sodium citrate tube. The WBC differential count and platelet count are obtained from the new specimen; however, the platelet count must be manually corrected for the 9:10 sodium citrate dilution by multiplying by 1.1. The rest of the CBC parameters are recorded from the K_2EDTA tube.

Cold Hemagglutinins

Cold hemagglutinins are IgM immunoglobulins that bind RBC antigens i and I at 4–6 °C. Most are harmless, although those that react at 30 °C to 37 °C may cause cold agglutinin disease with Raynaud phenomenon or hemolysis. Cold hemagglutinins may agglutinate RBCs in hematology specimens maintained at room temperature. The agglutination is non-diagnostic and generates implausibly high MCV and RDW results. RBC counts, HCT values, and WBC differential results cannot be trusted. The HGB, total WBC, and platelet counts may be accurate.

Agglutination may be dispersed by 15 *minutes' incubation at 37* °C followed by brief rocking or inversion. If this does not work, a fresh specimen is collected, transported, stored, and assayed immediately at 37 °C.

Rule of Three

Hematology laboratorians use the "*rule of three*" with each specimen to detect artifacts such as cold hemagglutinins and instrument malfunctions. The RBC count in millions/μL × 3 should approximate the hemoglobin in g/dL (HGB), and the HGB in g/dL × 3 should roughly equal the HCT in percent. If these rules are not met and the RBC morphology appears normal, the assay is repeated.

Specimens for Flow Cytometry

EDTA-anticoagulated whole blood and bone marrow specimens stored at room temperature, 18 °C to 24 °C, for up to 24 hours are used for flow cytometry (5). Bone marrow and tissue specimens in Hanks or RPMI can be used for flow up to four days.

Sedimentation Rate Specimens

Black-top evacuated glass tubes containing 3.8% sodium citrate are used for the erythrocyte sedimentation rate (ESR) test. The tubes provide a 1:5 dilution; 1 part anticoagulant to 4 parts whole blood, which is directly transferred to the ESR apparatus without further dilution (6).

The Complete Blood Count (CBC)

The CBC is the standard hematology profile. The specimen is accessioned and aspirated by an automated hematology analyzer, which provides the following assays, listed with reference intervals.

Table 1. RBC-Related Adult Reference Intervals (RIs)

RBC-Related Assays	Adult Male	Adult Female
Erythrocyte (red blood cell, RBC) count	4.4–5.8 million/µL	3.8–5.2 million/µL
Hematocrit (HCT)	39–50%	33–45%
Hemoglobin (HGB)	13.5–17.0 g/dL	11.3–15.2 g/dL

	Adults of Both Genders
Mean cell volume (MCV)	80–96 femtoliters (fL)
Mean cell hemoglobin concentration (MCHC)	32–36%
Mean cell hemoglobin (MCH)	27–33 picograms (pg)
Red cell distribution width (RDW)	11–16%
Absolute reticulocyte count (ARC) (7)	22,400–147,500/µL
Visual reticulocyte count (VRET%)	0.7–2.4%

Table 2. WBC- and Platelet-Related Adult RIs

WBCs and Platelet Count	Relative	Absolute
Total leukocyte (white blood cell, WBC) count		4,000–11,000/µL
Polymorphonuclear neutrophils (SEGs and BANDs)	35–84%	1,480–9,240/µL
Segmented neutrophils (SEGs)	35–73%	1,480–8,030/µL
Band neutrophils (BANDs)	0–11%	0–1,210/µL
Eosinophils (EOs)	0–5%	0–550/µL
Monocytes (MONOs)	4–13%	160–1,430/µL
Lymphocytes (LYMPHs)	10–44%	600–3,440/µL
Basophils (BASOs)	0–2%	0–220/µL
Platelet count		150,000–400,000/µL

*Pediatric RIs differ significantly and vary with age. See (7).

The laboratorian performs a *blood film examination* (BFE) whenever profiling instrument results fall outside selected action limits. Using a clinical grade microscope, the microscopist compares blood film WBC and platelet distributions to the instrument-generated WBC and platelet counts, and reviews and comments on the RBC morphology, comparing it to the indices MCV, MCHC, and RDW and to the reticulocyte parameters ARC and VRET%. The laboratorian systematically reviews, identifies, and tabulates WBCs, called a *WBC differential count*, expressing their distribution as a percentage and absolute count as shown in Table 2. Visual results should approximate instrument-generated WBC percentages and absolute counts; however, the visual review provides for identification of abnormalities the instrument is unable to detect. When a visual differential count is performed, the results are transcribed and supersede the instrument-generated results.

Histograms and Scattergrams

Hematology-profiling instruments provide frequency distributions of RBCs, WBCs, and platelets, called *histograms.* Frequency is plotted on the Y (vertical) scale and cell volume on the X (horizontal) scale. Histogram review assists the laboratorian in describing MCV, volume variation (RDW), and abnormal populations of cells (8).

RBC Histograms

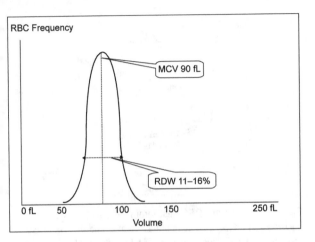

Figure 1. Normal RBC histogram. The RBC histogram ranges from 50 to 150 fL. The peak of the tracing represents the MCV, near 90 fL. The RDW expresses the coefficient of variation in RBC volume and is reflected in the broadness of the tracing. The distribution may have a slight skew to the right, representing RBC coincidence.

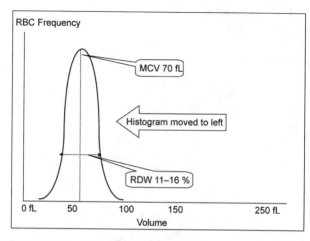

Figure 2. Microcytic RBC histogram. In the microcytic anemias such as iron deficiency anemia, thalassemia, and anemia of chronic disease, the distribution moves left with the peak or MCV in the range of 60 to 80 fL. The RDW may be normal or slightly increased, depending on the condition.

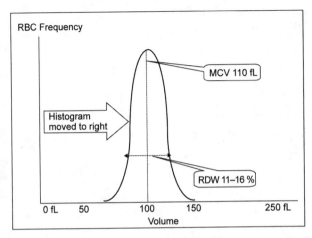

Figure 3. Macrocytic RBC histogram. In the macrocytic anemias, megaloblastic or refractory anemia, or in liver disease, the distribution moves right with the peak or MCV in the 100–120 fL range. The RDW is mildly increased.

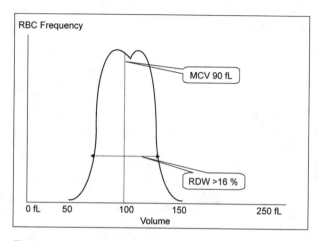

Figure 4. Bimodal RBC histogram. A dimorphic RBC pattern is reflected by a bimodal histogram with a markedly elevated RDW. Although the MCV may be normal at 90 fL, there are two RBC populations. This occurs early following therapy for iron deficiency anemia or megaloblastic anemia. It is also observed after transfusion or in sideroblastic or refractory anemia with ringed sideroblasts (RARS).

WBC Histograms and Scattergrams

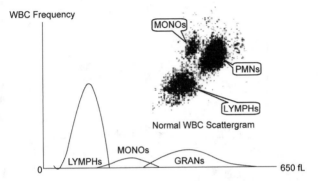

Figure 5. Normal WBC histogram. The WBC histogram scale ranges from 50 to 650 fL. Three peaks appear: LYMPHs, MONOs, and granulocytes (GRANs). GRANs include BANDs, SEGs, BASOs, and EOs. The histogram cannot independently be used to detect eosinophilia, basophilia, or an elevated BAND count, called a left shift.

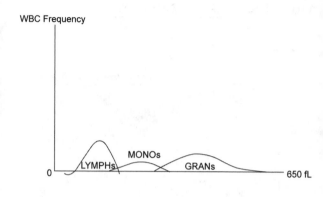

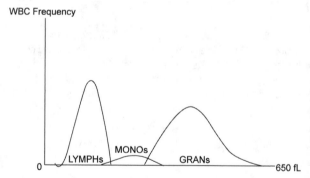

Figure 6. WBC histograms in lymphopenia and neutrophilia. The WBC histogram can strikingly illustrate lymphocytosis, lymphopenia, monocytosis, neutrophilia, and neutropenia. Lymphopenia, LYMPH count below 600/μL (top), and neutrophilia, GRAN count over 8,030/μL (bottom), are illustrated above.

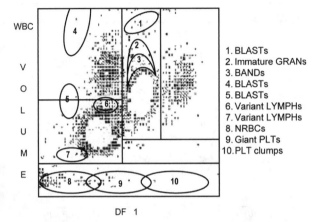

Figure 7. WBC Beckman-Coulter scattergram. High-end hematology profiling instruments provide *scattergrams* (scatterplots) that graph cell volume on the Y scale and a complexity characteristic such as laser light scatter on the X scale (cytoplasm granularity). Frequency is represented by distributions of color-coded dots. Circuitry adds thresholds that classify events as illustrated in the legend above. Instruments with scattergrams can separately delineate LYMPHs (lower left), MONOs (upper left), PMNs and BANDs, center, EOs, upper right, and BASOs, not visible. The instrument can also suggest, but not definitively identify, abnormal cells as listed in the legend.

Platelet Histograms

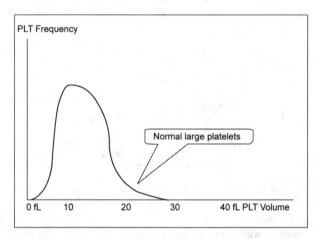

Figure 8. Platelet histogram. The platelet histogram ranges from 0 to 30 fL and is log-normal as the normal population contains a subset of right-skewed higher-volume platelets. Thrombocytopenia, thrombocytosis, and an increase in platelet volume are easily illustrated in the platelet histogram.

WBC Morphology in Wright-Stained Blood Films

When instrument parameters exceed established limits, laboratory professionals review blood films for abnormal WBC and RBC morphology. Morphologic changes are identified and graded based on their frequency and intensity, as slight (SLT, 1+), moderate (MOD, 2+), or marked (MKD, 3+, 4+) (9).

Polymorphonuclear neutrophils (PMNs) are either immature band-nucleus neutrophils (BANDs) or mature segmented nucleus neutrophils (SEGs). In acute inflammation, particularly bacterial infection, the SEG count exceeds 8,030/µL (73%), and the BAND count exceeds 1,210/µL (11%) in adults. The increase in bands is called "*left shift*" (10). In bacterial infections, the BANDs and SEGs appear *vacuolated* and display scattered dark primary granules called *toxic granulation*. *Döhle bodies* are 0.5 µm clear blue cytoplasmic islands, pathological accumulations of endoplasmic reticulum, that are less frequent but also support the diagnosis of infection or inflammation (11).

Lymphocytes (LYMPHs) appear nearly circular and mononuclear. *Variant LYMPHs, also called reactive LYMPHs, atypical LYMPHs, or Downey cells* have increased cytoplasm, abnormal cytoplasmic color distribution, and distorted nuclei. Variant LYMPHs often accompany LYMPH counts that exceed 3,440/µL (44%) in adults and signal viral infections, particularly with Epstein-Barr virus (infectious mononucleosis).

RBC Morphology in Wright-Stained Blood Films

Table 3. Variations in RBC Diameter

Term	Description	Association	RBC Index
Normocytic RBC	Orange biconcave disk with pale center, 6–7 µm diameter	Normal	MCV 80–96 fL
Macrocyte	Diameter >7 µm, often oval, center may not be pale	Macrocytosis in megaloblastic and refractory anemia, liver disease	MCV >96 fL
Microcyte	Diameter less than 6 µm, pale center is increased in diameter	Microcytic/ hypochromic anemias include iron deficiency anemia, anemia of chronic disease, and thalassemia	MCV <80 fL, MCHC <32%
Anisocytosis	Variation in RBC diameter	Broad distribution severe anemia. Dimorphic RBC pattern in recovering iron deficiency or megaloblastic anemia, transfusion, sideroblastic anemia	RDW >16%

Table 4. Variations in RBC Color

Term	Description	Association	RBC Index
Normochromic RBC	Orange biconcave disk with pale center, 6–7 µm diameter	Normal	MCHC 32–36%
Hypochromic RBC	Pale central zone increased in diameter though overall diameter is decreased	Microcytic/hypochromic anemias include iron deficiency anemia, anemia of chronic disease, and thalassemia	MCV <80 fL, MCHC <32%
Polychromic (polychromatophilic) RBC: polychromatophilia or polychromasia	Diameter >7 µm, bluish cytoplasm, no pale center	Bone marrow compensation in hemolytic anemia, comparable to reticulocytes in vital stain preparations	MCV normal or >96 fL, ARC exceeds 147,500/µL, VRET% >2.4%

There is no description or association for "hyperchromia" and the term is seldom used. An MCHC >36% indicates spherocytes, addressed in Table 5, "Variations in RBC shape."

Table 5. Variations in RBC Shape

Term/Synonyms	Description	Association
Stomatocyte	Pale center shaped like fish-mouth	Unreported artifact unless uniform, which then indicates *liver disease*
Echinocytes, burr cells, crenated cells	Regular pointed plasma membrane projections	Unreported artifact unless uniform, which then indicates *plasma pH or osmolality imbalance*

Table 5. (continued)

Term/Synonyms	Description	Association
Acanthocytes	Irregular pointed plasma membrane projections	Severe *lipid imbalance* or inherited abetalipoproteinemia
Ovalocyte, elliptocyte	Oval-shaped, often macrocytic	*Macro-ovalocytes* seen in megaloblastic and refractory anemia, ovalocytes with normal MCV indicate *hereditary ovalocytosis, elliptocytosis*
Spherocyte	Reduced diameter, no pale center	MCHC >36%. Seen in hereditary spherocytosis and warm autoimmune hemolytic anemia
Schistocyte, schizocyte, keratocyte, helmet cell	RBC fragment	Intravascular hemolysis, microangiopathic hemolytic anemia (MAHA) as in disseminated intravascular coagulation (DIC) or thrombotic thrombocytopenic purpura (TTP)
Drepanocyte, sickle cell	Sickle shape	Sickle cell disease in crisis
Codocyte, target cell	RBC with broad pale zone and "bulls-eye"	Sickle cell disease, thalassemia, refractory anemia, liver disease
Dacryocyte, teardrop cell	Single pointed projection	Myelofibrosis, extramedullary hematopoiesis (EMH), metastatic tumor in bone marrow
Poikilocytosis	Bizarre, unnamed shapes	Burns, pyropoikilocytosis, severe thalassemia, severe iron deficiency anemia

Table 6. RBC Inclusions

Term	Description	Association
Basophilic stippling, punctuate basophilia	Abundant evenly distributed regular dark blue specks, near visual resolution	Precipitated endoplasmic reticulum caused by heavy metal poisoning, megaloblastic and other anemias caused by abnormal RBC production
Howell-Jolly body	Single prominent dark blue particle	Nuclear fragment (DNA), splenectomy, megaloblastic and other anemias caused by abnormal RBC production
Cabot rings	Thin blue circle or figure "eight"	Spindle fibers. Megaloblastic and other anemias caused by abnormal RBC production
Pappenheimer bodies, siderotic granules in iron stain	Irregular dark blue particles, 4–6 per RBC, azure in Prussian blue iron stain	Precipitated hemosiderin RBCs are called siderocytes. Indicate abnormal iron metabolism as in sideroblastic or refractory anemia
Hemoglobin C crystals	Dark red intracellular "bar of gold," "Washington monument"	Hemoglobin C disease
Hemoglobin SC crystals	Dark red intracellular "gun" or "glove"	Compound heterozygous hemoglobin SC disease
Parasites	Signet ring, schizont, or gametes	Malaria: *Plasmodium sp*, Babesia: *Babesia sp*

Table 7. RBC Population Abnormalities

Term	Description	Association
Agglutination	Irregular RBC clumps visible at 100× magnification	IgM allo- or autoantibody. Transfusion reaction or cold agglutinin
Rouleaux	RBC clumps resembling "stack of coins," visible at low power	Plasma protein imbalance, M-protein in myeloma
Dimorphic population	RBCs of two diameters or two volumes (Figure 4)	Bimodal RBC histogram, RDW exceeding 16%. Recovering iron deficiency or megaloblastic anemia, transfusion, sideroblastic anemia.

Erythrocyte Sedimentation Rate (ESR)

The ESR reflects an underlying inflammatory process; elevated ESRs are seen in chronic inflammation, rheumatologic, and neoplastic conditions.

Effect of Plasma and RBCs on ESR

Elevated levels of fibrinogen and serum α-, β-, and γ-globulin raise the ESR. Severe anemia and macrocytes raise the ESR and microcytes, and severe poikilocytosis such as sickle cells retard the rate of RBC sedimentation.

Methods

Anticoagulated whole blood RBCs are allowed to settle in thin bore tubes. The interface of RBCs and plasma is compared to whole blood column height at 60 minutes.

- Westergren method uses a 150 mm whole blood column. It is the most common and uses citrated blood sample.
- Modified Westergren method uses EDTA blood and saline dilution.
- Micro-ESR using 200 µL whole blood and very thin bore tubes is useful in children.

Normal Ranges

- 0–10 mm/hour: males <50 years old
- 0–20 mm/hour: females <50 years old
- 30–40 mm/hour: >85 years old

Interpretation

Elevated ESRs are found in rheumatological conditions, impending sickle cell crisis, prostate cancer, and Hodgkin lymphoma. In lymphomas, higher levels at the time of diagnosis indicate poor prognosis. Accuracy is profoundly affected by specimen management and may be compromised by short draws and clots.

Serum Viscosity

Blood viscosity affects vascular flow; normal serum viscosity ranges from 1.4 to 1.8 *centipoises*. Viscosity greater than four centipoises is accompanied by vascular stasis and tissue hypoperfusion manifested by hyperviscosity syndrome: symptoms of dizziness and blurred vision. In fully established hyperviscosity syndrome, viscosity exceeds 5 centipoises.

Hyperviscosity is found in polycythemia vera, plasma cell dyscrasia, myeloma, and Waldenström macroglobulinemia. It is most often associated with elevated IgM, rarely with other myeloma proteins. Viscosity rises in leukocytosis >200,000/μL, as may develop in leukemia.

Bone Marrow Aspirate and Biopsy

Many hematological, infectious, and inflammatory disorders require *bone marrow aspirate and biopsy* review (12). A hematopathologist and a clinical laboratorian comprise the bone marrow collection team. The first step is to collect a peripheral blood sample to compare with the bone marrow specimen. The bone marrow aspirate and biopsy are next collected by the pathologist, usually from the posterior superior iliac crest. The aspirate is smeared on glass slides and stained with Wright stain. The biopsy is fixed and stained with a hematoxylin-eosin dye. Additional marrow aspirate may be preserved for culture, phenotyping, cytogenetics, and special stains as necessary.

Bone Marrow Aspirate

The bone marrow aspirate is readily available for examination after staining. The pathologist uses 100× total magnification to confirm cellularity and architecture and estimate megakaryocytes. There should be 3–5 megakaryocytes per low power field, though the count varies with the distribution and concentration of cells. Megakaryocyte report comments may include *normal, increased, decreased, decreased nuclear ploidy, increased nuclear ploidy, or megakaryocyte dysplasia.*

Malignant disorders may take on distinct patterns visible at 100×. *Sheets of immature cells, fields of unvaried blasts or mature cells, or clumped focal patterns* are clues for disease, to be confirmed using a higher power magnification. For example, multiple myeloma may be evidenced by sheets of abnormal plasma cells.

At 500× or 1000× total magnification, the pathologist looks for cell patterns in the areas surrounding bony spicules, asking the following questions:

- Do *megakaryocytes* appear to be producing platelets?
- Are all stages of *myelocytic and normoblastic* maturation present in the expected ratios?
- Is there a gap (*hiatus*) in any maturation sequence?
- Is the morphology of each cell lineage normal?
- What abnormal cells are present, and how abundant are they?

For confirmation, the pathologist may perform a *bone marrow differential by identifying* and tabulating 500 nucleated cells. The expected results are seen in Table 8.

Table 8. Normal Distribution of Bone Marrow Aspirate Cells

Cell	Reference Interval	Cell	Reference Interval
Myeloblasts	0.3–2.5%	Plasma cells	0–2%
Promyelocytes	1–8%	Histiocytes (reticulum cells)	0.2–2%
Myelocytes	5–21%	Rubriblasts (pronormoblasts)	0–1%
Metamyelocytes	6–22%	Prorubricytes	
BANDs	6–36%	(basophilic normoblasts)	0–3%
PMNs	9–27%	Rubricytes	
EOs	0–5%	(polychromic normoblasts)	3–9%
BASOs	0–1%	Metarubricytes	
MONOs	0–3%	(orthochromic normoblasts)	2–18%
LYMPHs	3–24%	Myeloid:erythroid (M:E)	
Variant LYMPHs	0%	ratio*	2–4:1

*Myeloid:erythroid ratio excludes lymphocytes, plasma cells, and histiocytes.

Bone Marrow Biopsy

The pathologist reviews the biopsy for *bone marrow anatomy (architecture) and cellularity*. The marrow of a 50-year-old should be *approximately 50% cellular hematopoietic tissue*; the remainder is adipocytes and fibrous tissue. Cellularity is the inverse of age and varies by 10% for each ten years; thus a 40-year-old's cellularity should be approximately 60% and a 60-year-old's, about 40%. Cellularity comments may include "*normocellular, hypocellular, acellular, hypercellular, or packed marrow*." A number of hematological diseases affect the localization of hematopoietic cells, and any disturbance to the normal architecture is evidence for disease (13,14).

Table 9. Indications for Bone Marrow Examination

Neoplastic	Primary diagnosis of acute leukemias and myeloproliferative disorders
	Diagnosis and staging of Hodgkin or non-Hodgkin lymphomas and hemophagocytic syndromes
	Myelodysplastic syndromes, mast cell disease, metastatic tumors
Marrow failures	Hypoplastic or aplastic anemia, myelodysplastic syndromes
	Suspected marrow necrosis secondary to tumor or severe infections such as Parvovirus or others
	Pure red cell aplasia (PRCA), severe thrombocytopenia to delineate immune from amegakaryocytic
	Sickle cell crisis, idiosyncratic drug-induced marrow suppression
Post-treatment	Post-chemotherapy marrow assessment to determine marrow recovery and minimal residual disease (MRD)
Infections	Peripheral blood cultures and polymerase chain reaction are more useful; however, bone marrow biopsy may be necessary to exclude infiltrative processes or fibrosis

Contra-indications	Severe coagulation factor deficiency such as hemophilia. Low platelet count is not absolute contraindication
Sites	Posterior or anterior iliac crest for aspirate and biopsy, sternum for aspirate only, and proximal tibia in infants, for aspirate only

Specimens

Peripheral blood	Air-dried, fixed, and Wright-Giemsa-stained films are essential to correlate with bone marrow findings. CBC, RBC morphology, WBC differentials, and platelet morphology complement marrow examination. In addition, flow cytometry, cytogenetic analysis, and molecular studies can be performed if blasts or atypical cells are present in the blood.
Bone marrow aspirate	0.5–2.0 mL collected in a syringe. Part of the specimen is used for making air-dried *marrow smears*. Marrow aspirate is most suited for flow cytometry, cytogenetic analysis, fluorescent in situ hybridization (FISH), and molecular studies. If aspirate was not obtainable (dry tap), an extra bone marrow biopsy may be submitted in RPMI-1640 for later tissue disaggregation for these studies. Excess aspirate is fixed in formalin and submitted for clot sections.
Bone marrow biopsy	1.0–1.5 cm core biopsy is required. Immediate "touch imprints" "touch imprints" of the biopsy are extremely useful in assessing cellular morphology. After imprints are made, the biopsy specimen is fixed in neutral buffered 10% formalin for 2–3 hours, decalcified, and processed in the histology laboratory. Hematoxylin and eosin (H&E) stained sections and appropriate cytochemical and immunohistochemistry stains are performed.

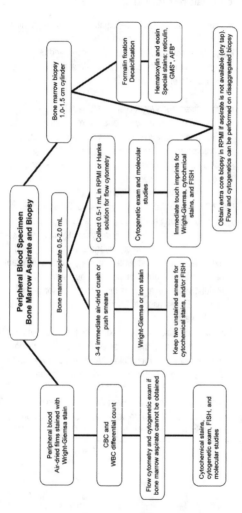

FISH, fluorescent in situ hybridization; GMS, Gomori-methenamine stain; AFB, acid fast bacilli stain.

Figure 9. Bone marrow aspirate and biopsy algorithm.

26

Anemia

Anemia is one of the most common conditions encountered in clinical practice. It may be caused by blood loss; iron, B_{12}, and folate deficiency states; inherited enzyme and membrane defects; and destruction through autoimmune and angiopathic hemolysis.

Table 10. Most Common Causes of Anemia

Anemia Categories	Worldwide Incidence
Iron deficiency	38%
Thalassemias (α and β) and sickle cell disease	36%
Anemia of chronic disease (ACD)	17%
Autoimmune hemolytic anemia, enzyme defects, membrane defects, and aplastic anemia	<7%
B_{12} or folate deficiency	~1%
Other miscellaneous causes	<1%

Table 11. RBC Production Deficiencies (see Figure 10)

Types	Causes
Nutrition	Iron, B_{12}, or folate deficiency
Marrow suppression	Anemia of chronic disease (ACD) and toxic conditions
	Viral suppression such as parvovirus infection
	Drugs: chemotherapy and idiosyncratic response
Myelophthisic	Replacement of marrow by fibrosis, tumor, acute or chronic leukemia, or granulomas
Lack of stem cells	Hypoplastic or aplastic anemia
Hemophagocytosis	Acquired hemophagocytic syndrome with pancytopenia in children

Table 12. Iron Metabolism (see Figure 11)

Compartments	Iron, mg	%
Hemoglobin	1,750–2,000	67
Storage: ferritin		
and hemosiderin	400–1,000	27
Myoglobin	250–350	3.5
Cellular labile pool		
(LIP*, cytoplasmic bound iron)	80	2.2
Other tissues	8	0.2
Transport iron	3	0.08

These are estimates for a person weighing 70 kg (data from many sources).
*LIP: labile iron pool.

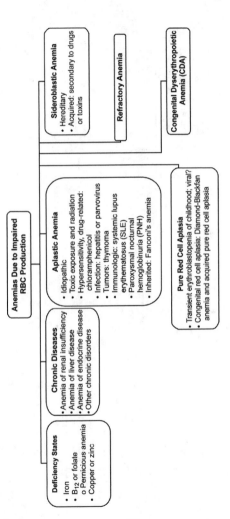

Anemias Due to Impaired RBC Production

Deficiency States
- Iron
- B₁₂ or folate
  - o Pernicious anemia
- Copper or zinc

Chronic Diseases
- Anemia of renal insufficiency
- Anemia of liver disease
- Anemia of endocrine disease
- Other chronic disorders

Aplastic Anemia
- Idiopathic
- Toxic exposure and radiation
- Hypersensitivity, drug-related: chloramphenicol
- Infection: hepatitis or parvovirus
- Tumors: thymoma
- Immunologic: systemic lupus erythematosus (SLE)
- Paroxysmal nocturnal hemoglobinuria (PNH)
- Inherited: Fanconi's anemia

Sideroblastic Anemia
- Hereditary
- Acquired: secondary to drugs or toxins

Refractory Anemia

Pure Red Cell Aplasia
- Transient erythroblastopenia of childhood; viral?
- Congenital red cell aplasia: Diamond-Blackfan anemia and acquired pure red cell aplasia

Congenital Dyserythropoietic Anemia (CDA)

Figure 10. Differentiating anemias caused by impaired RBC production.

29

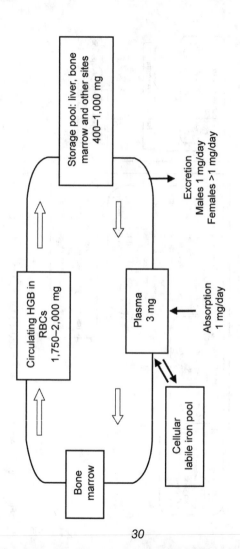

Figure 11. Iron metabolism.

Iron Deficiency Anemia

Iron Absorption and Incorporation into The Erythroblast

Absorption of iron from the GI tract is an active process in two phases:

- *Luminal* iron receptors are present on the mucosal surface of the duodenum and proximal small intestine. Heme iron is absorbed more rapidly than non-heme iron (15).

- *Mucosal:* Transport across the mucosal wall is facilitated by *hem-transporter* for heme-iron and *divalent metal transporter* (DMT-1) for non-heme iron. Intracellular mucosal ferritin and membrane proteins *ferroprotein-1* and *hephaestin* deliver iron to plasma transferrin. This uptake is modulated by body iron needs. A negative regulatory mechanism operates through *hepcidin,* which inhibits iron absorption into the duodenum and inhibits release of macrophage iron in the bone marrow (16).

Plasma transport: The plasma transports approximately 3 mg of iron with a turnover rate >10 times in 24 hours. Iron from different pools is exchanged through plasma (17).

- *Transferrin* is the major plasma iron transport protein, an 80-KD glycoprotein synthesized in macrophages and the liver. It delivers iron to tissues throughout the body and to marrow erythroblasts by binding erythroblast transferrin receptor CD71. Each transferrin molecule can bind two iron ions, and 25–35% of total plasma transferrin is bound to iron.

- *Total iron-binding capacity (TIBC) or % transferrin saturation* assays measure the plasma transferrin capacity by saturating available binding sites *in vitro*. Transport iron is a labile pool subject to diurnal variations. Additionally, transferrin levels fluctuate in liver disease and other inflammatory conditions. Consequently, plasma transferrin and TIBC are poor measures of total iron stores, particularly unreliable in liver disease.

- *Incorporation of iron into erythroblasts:* The CD71 receptor-transferrin complex is incorporated into the erythroblast by endocytosis. Erythroblasts have more receptors than their more differentiated erythroid precursors and incorporate 80–90% of the iron into hemoglobin.
- *Free erythrocyte protoporphyrin (FEP):* Protoporphyrin IX accumulates in erythrocyte cytoplasm when iron is not incorporated into hemoglobin such as in *iron deficiency, lead poisoning, and ferrochelatase deficiency*.

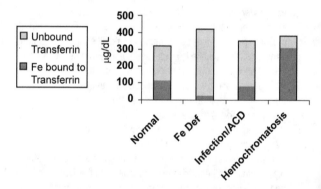

Figure 12. Concentration of transferrin and transferrin-bound iron in three conditions.
ACD, anemia of chronic disease

Causes of Iron Deficiency

- *Inadequate intake* is the most common cause of iron deficiency. Even in developed countries, most diets of women of
  childbearing age are inadequate to keep mothers and infants
  in positive iron balance. At least 20% of pre-menopausal
  women have slightly depleted iron stores, and 3% are anemic.
  Iron diversion to the fetus for erythropoiesis, and bleeding at
  delivery account for the loss of about 900 mg, equivalent to two
  liters of blood. Lactation accounts for another 30 mg of iron
  loss per month.

- *Adult-acquired iron deficiency:* chronic blood loss from the GI
  tract is the most common cause of iron deficiency in men and
  post-menopausal women. This may be due to peptic ulcer disease, gastritis, hemorrhoids, and vascular anomalies. Aspirin and
  other non-steroidal anti-inflammatory drugs (NSAIDs), steroids,
  and alcohol frequently cause gastritis and may account for mild
  continuous GI bleeding.

- *Malignancy* accounts for 5% of all adult GI bleeds; among the eld-
  erly, the risk is higher. *Always work up iron deficiency in adults;*
  GI polyps and colon carcinoma are the most common causes for
  GI bleeding in the elderly.

- *Malabsorption* of iron is relatively uncommon. It is seen after partial gastrectomy, duodenal resection, celiac disease (non-tropical
  sprue), and parasitic infestation (intestinal helminthiasis).

- *Iron deficiency at birth* may be caused by fetomaternal hemorrhage, twin-to-twin transfusion, fetal hematomas, amniocentesis,
  and premature umbilical cord clamping.

- *Intravascular hemolysis* from a variety of causes can result in iron loss. Mechanical destruction of circulating RBCs known as *march hemoglobinuria* is seen in athletes and in patients with prosthetic heart valves, where it is called the "Waring blender" syndrome. In *paroxysmal nocturnal hemoglobinuria* (PNH), patients have episodic hemolysis with urinary loss of iron. Sickle cell anemia and thalassemia both have a hemolytic component that may also lead to iron deficiency.

- Other causes of iron loss are *disseminated intravascular coagulation* (DIC) and *thrombotic thrombocytopenic purpura* (TTP) due to brisk intravascular hemolysis.

- Phlebotomy for laboratory tests: Patients may lose *more than 50 mL/day* for repeat arterial blood gas assays, CBCs, clinical chemistry, enzyme profiles, and many other laboratory tests.

Clinical Findings in Iron Deficiency

In the initial stages of iron deficiency, iron stores are reduced but there are no symptoms. Once anemia is established at a HGB <8 g/dL, multiple signs and symptoms appear: weakness, lassitude, and exertional dyspnea. Other signs include mucosal pallor, angular stomatitis, glossitis, koilonychia (spoon-shaped nails), gastric atrophy, and menorrhagia.

Laboratory Investigation of Iron Deficiency

- *Complete blood count:* low HGB, HCT, RBC count, MCV, and MCHC. The peripheral blood film is a quick screening tool to detect iron deficiency anemia and thalassemia by observing microcytic hypochromic RBCs. Anemia of chronic disease, sometimes associated with microcytic hypochromic RBCs, needs to be ruled out. Bone marrow exam is not indicated to confirm iron deficiency.

- *Serum ferritin:* this is the most reliable assay as it directly reflects body iron stores. Normal range is 33–350 ηg/mL. In normal individuals, 1 ηg/mL serum ferritin roughly represents 8–10 mg of storage iron. Levels below 10 ηg/mL are diagnostic of iron deficiency. However, in certain chronic conditions such as liver disease, normal to high ferritin levels may mask iron deficiency.
- *Serum iron:* this is iron bound to transferrin. Normal range is 60–160 μg/dL. Iron levels fluctuate widely and may not reflect body iron stores. High levels are seen in sideroblastic and hemolytic anemias.
- *TIBC or % saturation:* reflects measurement of serum transferrin by saturating available binding sites. Normally 25–35% of transferrin is saturated with iron. In iron deficiency, transferrin synthesis is increased with lower saturation (<10%). Because serum iron and transferrin values fluctuate, % saturation is more clinically significant than either value alone. In iron overload conditions, TIBC is decreased as transferrin is >80% saturated.

Table 13. Normal and Iron Deficiency Laboratory Parameters

Test	Normal	Tissue Iron Depletion	Iron Deficiency Erythropoiesis	Severe Anemia
Iron stores by bone marrow iron stain	1–3+	None detected	None detected	None detected
Serum ferritin	33–350 ng/mL	<12 ng/mL	<12 ng/mL	<12 ng/mL
Serum iron	60–160 µg/dL	<100 µg/dL	<60 µg/dL	<40 µg/dL
TIBC/transferrin levels	300 µg/dL	>300 µg/dL	>300 µg/dL	>450 µg/dL
Transferrin saturation	33%	33%	>20%	<10%
HGB	Males: 13.5–17.0 g/dL Females: 11.3–15.2 g/dL	Normal	9–12 g/dL	<8 g/dL
MCV	80–96 fL	Normal	80–85 fL	<80 fL
MCHC	32–36%	Normal	Normal	<30%
RDW	<16%	Normal	>16%	>16%
Free erythrocyte protoporphyrin (FEP)	30–70 µg/dL	70 µg/dL	>100 µg/dL	>100 µg/dL

Megaloblastic Anemia: Folate and Vitamin B_{12} Deficiency

Natural Distribution of B_{12} and Folate

Folates are widely distributed in nature and are synthesized by plants and microorganisms. Leafy vegetables, fruit, yeast, and liver and kidney meat are rich sources. Folates are heat-labile and destroyed by prolonged cooking. The minimum daily requirement is 50 μg; the adult recommended daily intake is approximately 100 μg, and during pregnancy, 500 μg.

Vitamin B_{12} (cyanocobalamin, Cbl) is produced only by microorganisms and is an absolute dietary requirement for humans. Animal proteins serve as the major B_{12} source: meat, cheese, milk and eggs. Legumes are a non-animal source. Vitamin B_{12} is heat-stable and survives cooking. The minimum daily requirement is 1.3 μg and B_{12} is stored well in tissues.

Vitamin B_{12} Metabolism

Absorption: B_{12} dissociates from food in low stomach pH. Free B_{12} is bound preferentially to high-affinity R-proteins (apo-R protein), forming a holo-R protein. This complex passes into the duodenum where pancreatic proteases cleave holo-R, releasing the B_{12} that subsequently binds intrinsic factor (IF), a glycoprotein synthesized by the parietal cells in the fundus.

Transport: The IF-B_{12} complex passes to the ileum, where it is bound by membrane-associated IF receptors, endocytosed, and degraded. B_{12} subsequently appears in the portal circulation bound to transcobalamin II, where it is transported to cellular sites.

Intracellular vitamin B_{12}: More than 95% of cellular B_{12} is bound to methylmalonic CoA mutase (MMCoA mutase) or methionine synthetase

(Me-Cbl), both of which catalyze intramolecular exchange of *one-carbon atom moieties*. For example, Me-Cbl transfers methyl groups from Me-B_{12} to homocysteine to form methionine.

Molecular Basis of Megaloblastic Changes

Vitamin B_{12} and folate deficiency: In B_{12} or folate deficiency, a net decrease in 5,10-methylene H4PteGlu interrupts the thymidylate synthetase-mediated conversion of dUMP to dTMP. The resulting block leads to decreased dTTP synthesis and the formation of excess dUTP. The dUTP is abnormally incorporated into DNA, resulting in nuclear dissociation called karyorrhexis and cell death.

In the bone marrow, *defective DNA synthesis* is reflected in arrest of nuclear maturation, increased cells in the G2 phase of the cell cycle, and a mix of cells with 2N and 4N ploidy. Meanwhile, *RNA maturation and cytoplasmic organelle production* remains normal, leading to *nuclear-cytoplasmic asynchrony*. Additionally, there is *intramedullary hemolysis*, raising plasma LDH levels secondary to cell cycle arrest and karyorrhexis.

Rapidly dividing non-hematopoietic cells are also affected. Epithelial cells lining the buccal mucosa, tongue, and other parts of the GI tract and squamous epithelial cells of the skin show visible changes. B_{12} deficiency results in severe *neurological changes* characterized by patchy demyelination and axonal degeneration, leading to cerebral abnormalities and subacute combined degeneration of the spinal cord.

Clinical Findings in Megaloblastic Anemia

Usual onset of megaloblastic anemia is insidious, progressing so slowly that the patient adapts and consequently first presents with severe anemia. Findings may include a low grade fever, glossitis, congestive heart failure, and neurological symptoms including loss of position sense, weakness, and neuropathy. There is no correlation between the degree of anemia and the presence of neurologic symptoms.

CBC, Bone Marrow, and Other Laboratory Findings

Look for an MCV exceeding 115 fL, with macro-ovalocytes and hypersegmented PMNs on the blood film. All marrow cell lineages are affected. Megaloblastic changes are seen in erythroblasts, resulting in diffuse punctate "cut salami" chromatin. Myelocytic maturation produces giant metamyelocytes and bands. Giant megakaryocytes also form. Serum LDH levels often exceed 1,000 U/L, especially in B_{12} deficiency, signaling ineffective erythropoiesis and hemolysis with cellular phagocytosis.

Table 14. B_{12} and Folate Deficiency Laboratory Tests

Test	Normal	Folate Deficiency	B_{12} Deficiency
Urine methylmalonic acid	<9 mg/24 hr	Normal	Increased
Deoxyuridine (DU) suppression	Normal	Abnormal	Abnormal
Urine FIGlu excretion	<17 mg/8 hr	Increased	Increased
Plasma homocysteine	<22 μmol/L	Increased	Increased
Serum B_{12}	>160 ηg/L	Normal or low	<50 ηg/L
Serum folate*	>6 μg/L	Low	Normal or increased
RBC folate*	>166 μg/L	Low	Low

*Serum folate fluctuates widely and rises after meals. Low serum folate levels are found in pregnancy and alcoholic liver disease. The RBC folate level is a more reliable indicator of tissue folate stores. RBC folate levels are more stable because the reduced form of tetrahydrofolate resides inside the cells.

The deoxyuridine (DU) suppression test detects impaired DU methylation and is a sensitive indicator of B_{12} and folate deficiency.

Anemia of Chronic Disease (ACD)

ACD is the most common anemia in hospitalized patients. RBC production is reduced in chronic diseases due to reduced erythropoiesis and impaired iron utilization. Reduced erythropoietin production secondary to interleukin-1 and tumor necrosis factor (TNF) is the hypothesized mechanism. Further, the liver secretes *hepcidin*, inhibiting iron absorption.

Table 15. Conditions Associated With ACD

Chronic microbial infections	Osteomyelitis and bacterial infections
Immune disorders	Rheumatoid arthritis and chronic inflammatory bowel disease
Malignancies	Carcinomas, Hodgkin and non-Hodgkin lymphomas

Laboratory Findings in ACD

Microcytic hypochromic RBCs with reduced MCV and MCHC may mimic iron deficiency or thalassemia. Low serum iron, reduced TIBC, and *reduced transferrin* with abundant iron stores in marrow macrophages.

Aplastic Anemia

Aplastic anemia is a hypo-productive state in which RBCs, WBCs, and platelets are reduced and the marrow is markedly hypocellular. Although the etiology is poorly understood, there are known associations with exposure to drugs called idiosyncratic reactions, dose-related responses to chemicals and toxins, and also stem cell defects and viral agents. Anemia may occur at any age, and the clinical course ranges from mild to severe. A CBC and bone marrow biopsy are used for diagnosis. Typically, two hypocellular bone marrow biopsies spaced over an 8–10 week interval are needed to confirm the diagnosis.

Marrow Failure

Pure red cell aplasia, also called *transient erythroblastopenia of childhood*, is seen only in children. The condition is related to viral illness and in most cases there is spontaneous recovery. In adults, pure red cell aplasia is immune-mediated and in some cases is secondary to thymoma.

Myelophthisic pancytopenia is caused by space-occupying lesions in the marrow, such as leukemia, metastatic tumors, or granulomas.

In some cases of *myelofibrosis, a leukoerythroblastic picture* that includes nucleated RBCs and early myeloid precursors is seen in the peripheral blood.

Myelodysplastic syndromes (MDS) may also progress to marrow failure with severe cytopenias and transfusion dependency.

Other rare conditions associated with marrow failure include *congenital dyserythropoietic anemia (CDA), and hereditary or acquired sideroblastic anemias.*

Hemoglobinopathies and Thalassemias

Normal Hemoglobin

Normal adult hemoglobin is a *tetramer* consisting of four globin chains: two α-chains and two β-chains, $\alpha_2\beta_2$. Each globin chain binds one heme molecule supporting a ferrous ion, Fe^{++}. The heme-Fe^{++} pocket transports a molecule of oxygen. Other normal chains are δ-globin, which is found in place of β-globin in hemoglobin A_2 ($\alpha_2\delta_2$), and γ-globin, which makes up fetal hemoglobin, HGB F ($\alpha_2\gamma_2$).

Globin gene expression is codominant. The α chains are composed of 141 amino acids; β, δ, and γ chains are 146 each. The genes for β, δ, and γ are located on chromosome 2, and for α, on chromosome 16. Globin chain production occurs in ribosomes of nucleated RBCs and reticulocytes (polychromic RBCs); mature RBCs lack mRNA and cannot produce globins.

Hemoglobinopathies are *qualitative* globin chain abnormalities and thalassemias are *quantitative* deficiencies.

Table 16. Normal Globin Chain Distribution

Adult Hemoglobins	Distribution	Globin Chains
HGB A_1	95–98%	$\alpha_2\beta_2$
HGB A_2	2.5–3.2%	$\alpha_2\delta_2$
HGF F (fetal)	0.8–2.0%	$\alpha_2\gamma_2$
HGB F distribution in children		
Newborns*	50–80%	
6 months	8%	
>6 months	1–2%	

*Varies with gestational age.

Globin Chain Embryology

- HGB A$_1$: $\alpha_2\beta_2$
  Synthesis of α and β chains begins in the second month of gestation; α synthesis exceeds β. Adult A$_1$ HGB production rises after birth to more than 95% by 3–6 months.
- HGB F: $\alpha_2\gamma_2$
  Synthesis of γ chains begins in the first month of gestation and rapidly increases to just before birth. Newborn hemoglobin is 50–80% HGB F. HGB F has slightly higher affinity for oxygen than HGB A. Production declines until the adult level of 1% HGB F is reached at 3–6 months.
- HGB A$_2$: $\alpha_2\delta_2$
  Synthesis of δ chains begins shortly before birth. The normal adult proportion of 2.5–3.2% HGB A$_2$ is reached at 3–6 months.
- Embryonic hemoglobins: These are synthesized before 3 months' gestation. Traces may be seen in normal newborns.

Table 17. Embryonic Hemoglobins

Embryonic Hemoglobin	Globin Chains
HGB Portland	$\zeta_2\gamma_2$
HGB Gower 1	$\zeta_2\varepsilon_2$
HGB Gower 2	$\alpha_2\varepsilon_2$

Oxygen Transport by Hemoglobin

Oxygen binds heme groups and is released to the tissues. The four heme groups sequentially bind O_2, altering the conformation of the hemoglobin molecule, called "heme-heme interaction," resulting in progressive increase of O_2 affinity. As the third and fourth heme groups deliver O_2 to the tissues, there is a progressive decrease in affinity, enhancing O_2 delivery.

Table 18. Partial Pressure and Percent Saturation of Oxygen

Location	Partial Pressure of Oxygen, pO_2	% Saturation
Lungs	100 mmHg	100%
Tissue	40 mmHg	66%

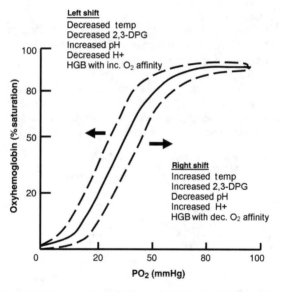

Figure 13. Oxygen dissociation curve. Molecules of 2,3 diphospho-glycerate (DPG, bisphosphoglycerate, BPG), H_2, CO_2, and ATP bind the central hemoglobin cavity and alter O_2-hemoglobin affinity. This generates a sigmoid O_2-hemoglobin dissociation curve.

Quantitatively and Functionally Abnormal Hemoglobins

There are at least 350 hemoglobin mutations or polymorphisms. Most have no physiologic significance. Here are examples of pathological hemoglobins and their genetic causes:

- Hemoglobins created by point mutations or by frame or terminator codon misreading:
  - HGB S: $\beta^{6Glu \rightarrow Val}$: valine is substituted for glutamine at the sixth position of the β-chain. When deoxygenated, HGB S forms insoluble linear crystals that distort RBCs into sickle shape, occluding vessels and causing hemolysis.
  - HGB C: $\beta^{6Glu \rightarrow Lys}$: lysine is substituted for glutamine at the sixth position of the β-chain. Viscous HGB C forms blunt crystals shaped like the Washington monument, reducing RBC deformability and causing hemolysis.
  - HGB Constant Spring: elongated α-globin chain
  - HGB Wayne: α-chain frame shift
- Hemoglobins created by unequal crossovers
  - HGB Lepore: δβ fusion with N and C terminal abnormalities
  - HGB Miyada: Lepore-like δβ fusion
- High oxygen affinity hemoglobins
  - HGB Chesapeake: an α-chain abnormality associated with mild polycythemia
- Low oxygen affinity hemoglobins
  - HGB Kansas: a β-chain abnormality that impairs oxygen uptake, resulting in cyanosis and anemia
- Unstable hemoglobins that precipitate in RBCs as Heinz bodies; more than 100 variants
  - HGB Hammersmith

Table 19. Relative Levels of HGBs A$_2$ F, H, S, and C in Various Hemoglobinopathies and Thalassemias

Disorder	HGB A$_1$	HGB A$_2$	HGB F	HGB H	HGB S	HGB C
β-Thalassemia minor	84–94%	4–5.8%	2–5%			
β-Thalassemia major	5–95%	5–7%	10–90%			
α-Thalassemia minor or trait	92–94%	2.5–3.2%				
HGB H disease (α-thalassemia intermedia or major)	60–75%	<2%		25–40%		
Homozygous sickle cell (HGB S) disease			15%		70–98%	
Homozygous HGB C disease			2–10%			90–98%
Heterozygous hereditary persistence of HGB F (HPFH)	62–92%	2.5–3.2%	5–35%			
Homozygous hereditary persistence of HGB F (HPFH)			100%			

Pathophysiology of the Hemoglobinopathies

- Intra- and extravascular (splenic) hemolysis
- Autosplenectomy
- Ischemic leg ulcers and infections
- Bone deformities
- Renal papillary necrosis
- Dactylitis
- Leg ulcers
- Crises
  - Veno-occlusive
  - Acute pulmonary with bilateral infiltrates
  - Splenic sequestration with acute splenomegaly, especially in childhood
  - Aplastic crises with extramedullary hematopoiesis and hepatosplenomegaly

Laboratory Tests for the Detection of Hemoglobinopathies

- Sodium dithionite solubility (Sickledex®): screen for HGB S; HCT must be at least 20%
  - Positive in sickle cell disease and trait, negative in HGB C disease or trait
- Hemoglobin electrophoresis at acid and alkaline pH: see Figure 14
- Globin chain electrophoresis
- Isoelectric focusing electrophoresis
- Heat or isopropanol stability tests for unstable hemoglobins
- O_2-HGB dissociation curve or venous blood gas assay for hemoglobins with high or low O_2 affinity
- Two dimension "fingerprinting" chromatography
- Gene mapping

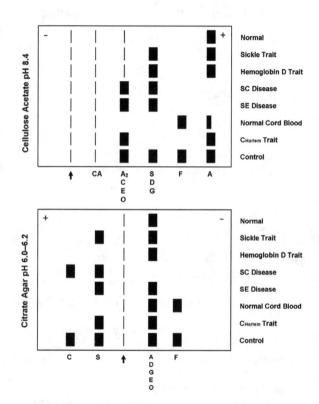

Figure 14. Anticipated hemoglobin electrophoresis results for alkaline cellulose acetate and acid citrate agar media.

CA, carbonic anhydrase; arrows indicate point of specimen application (18).

Thalassemia: Reduced α- or β-Globin Synthesis: α-Thalassemia, β-Thalassemia

- *Hypochromic microcytic* RBCs with markedly reduced MCV and MCHC
- Relative excess of alternate unsuppressed chain production results in *Heinz body precipitation,* membrane damage and hemolysis. For example, in α-thalassemia, unsuppressed β-chain synthesis produces β_4 tetramers, called HGB H, which precipitate on the inner surface of the cell membrane.
- Ineffective bone marrow erythropoiesis with high LDH

α-Thalassemias

- The most common thalassemias, caused by α-gene deletions.
- Each human has two (duplicated) maternal and two paternal α-genes.
- A single-gene deletion ($-\alpha/\alpha\alpha$) produces a *silent carrier* called α-thalassemia silent who may have no anemia but slight microcytosis and a very slight decrease in α/non-α chain production ratio.
- A two-gene deletion, α-thalassemia minor or intermedia, either *trans* ($-\alpha/-\alpha$) or *cis* ($--/\alpha\alpha$), causes mild anemia, though more severe in the Asian type. There are traces of HGB Bart's (γ_4) in the newborn or HGB H (β_4) in adults.
- A three-gene deletion ($--/-\alpha$) causes marked anemia and abundant HGB Bart's in the newborn or HGB H in adults, called HGB H disease.
- Hydrops fetalis: four-gene deletion with 100% HGB Bart's is lethal. The fetus dies in utero at term.
- Elongated α-chain: HGB Constant Spring

β-Thalassemias

- Defective conversion from heterogeneous nuclear β-chain RNA (hnRNA) to mRNA because of intron transcription errors
  - Normal β chains may be present
  - The β-thalassemia gene is designated β^+
  - Neither the γ nor the δ chains are affected, so HGB F and A_2 may be increased
- mRNA absent due to β-gene deletion or severely decreased due to defective β-gene transcription
  - The β-thalassemia gene is designated β^0

Other Thalassemias and Related Disorders

- Hereditary persistence of fetal hemoglobin (HPFH) with elevated HGB F
  - Distribution of HGB F in RBCs may be uniform or non-uniform
  - When combined with β-thalassemia, distribution is non-uniform
  - Symptoms are mild due to increased HGB F O_2 affinity
  - Detectable using the Kleihauer-Betke acid stain
- Variant globins: HGB Kenya, Lepore, and Miyada
- δβ-thalassemia lacks β and δ-chains so only HGB F is present

Double Heterozygous States

- Sickle cell/β-thalassemia S/β^+: symptoms are milder than sickle cell disease (SS)
- Sickle cell/β-thalassemia S/β^0: symptoms are similar to sickle cell disease (SS)
- HGB C/β-thalassemia C/β^+ or C/β^0: few symptoms

Laboratory Tests for Thalassemias

- Hypochromic microcytic RBCs and MCV and MCHC that may be markedly reduced
- Target cells may be prominent
- Hemoglobin electrophoresis to detect HGBs H, Bart's, F, and elevated A_2
- Kleihauer-Betke acid stain for fetal hemoglobin (uniform or non-uniform RBC staining)
- Globin chain synthesis rate: measures radiolabeled amino acids in reticulocytes
- Flow cytometry assay for fetal hemoglobin

Hemoglobin Byproducts

- *Methemoglobin (hemiglobin, Hi)* is produced by oxidation of heme iron from ferrous (Fe^{++}) to ferric (Fe^{+++}) valence state, which is unable to bind oxygen. Increased amounts manifest as chocolate brown discoloration of blood, and overt cyanosis when Hi exceeds 10% of the total hemoglobin. Hereditary Hi forms occur due to lack of NADH-cytochrome-b and an abnormal structure, HGB M, is reported. Secondary Hi arises from exposures to chemicals or drugs, for example, nitrites, chlorate, and quinones.
- *Sulfhemoglobin:* Sulfur is incorporated into hemoglobin during oxidative hemolysis, yielding partially oxidized and denatured hemoglobin. Heinz bodies, precipitates of denatured hemoglobin, may form on RBC membranes. Sulfhemoglobin cannot transport oxygen and small amounts are reported in patients receiving sulfonamides or aromatic amines.
- *Carboxyhemoglobin (HGB CO)* reflects high affinity for carbon monoxide (CO). Even 0.02% CO leads to a progressive increase.

HGB CO prevents the release of oxygen to the tissues as the oxygen dissociation curve is left-shifted, resulting in severe tissue anoxia. Mild chronic CO poisoning is not uncommon in busy streets, due to automobile emissions.

Hemolytic Anemias

Acute or chronic hemolytic anemia is caused by *accelerated destruction of circulating RBCs*. The magnitude of signs and symptoms is proportional to the rate of hemolysis. Hemolysis is suspected when there is *reduced HGB, HCT, and RBC count, jaundice, and an elevated reticulocyte count*. In severe cases, there may be nucleated red blood cells (NRBCs) in the peripheral blood. Leukocytosis and thrombocytosis are common findings in acute hemolysis as the myeloid stem cell that generates RBCs also differentiates into granulocytes and platelets. Other findings are elevated unconjugated (indirect) bilirubin, elevated lactate dehydrogenase (LDH), and reduced or absent haptoglobin. The full constellation of findings varies with the cause of the hemolytic anemia and, in particular, whether hemolysis is *intravascular or extravascular*.

Intravascular Hemolysis

Intravascular hemolysis (RBC rupture and release of hemoglobin into the blood vessel) may be *immune or non-immune*. An ABO mismatched hemolytic transfusion reaction, for example, causes acute *alloimmune* intravascular hemolysis. Naturally occurring IgM anti-A or anti-B antibodies bind the mismatched cell membrane, activate complement, and cause hemolysis via insertion of the membrane attack complex (MAC). Severe hemoglobinemia and hemoglobinuria ensue; these may lead to disseminated intravascular coagulation (DIC) and acute tubular necrosis. An acute hemolytic transfusion reaction may be rapidly fatal. Non-immune intravascular hemolysis may be caused by intracorpuscular RBC disorders or a variety of extracorpuscular factors as seen in Table 20.

Table 20. Conditions that Cause Non-Immune Hemolytic Anemias with Corresponding Laboratory Assays Used to Confirm the Diagnosis

Defect	Assays
Intracorpuscular: Membrane disorders	
Relatively common (1/5000): Hereditary spherocytosis (HS); hereditary elliptocytosis (HE, ovalocytosis)	Blood film RBC morphology with spherocytes or elliptocytes (ovalocytes); increased osmotic fragility test result; family studies; membrane protein electrophoresis
Rare: Hereditary pyropoikilocytosis (HPP); hereditary stomatocytosis (HST); hereditary xerocytosis; abetaliproteinemia-acanthocytosis; lecithin-cholesterol acyltransferase deficiency with codocytosis	Blood film RBC morphology with poikilocytes
Intracorpuscular: Hereditary enzyme deficiencies	
Glucose-6-phosphate dehydrogenase (G6PD) deficiency; pyruvate kinase deficiency; methemoglobin reductase deficiency	Oxidative denaturation of hemoglobin produces Heinz bodies detectable by supravital staining (new methylene blue or crystal violet); colorimetric and fluorescent spot screens for G6PD; G6PD enzyme assay; fluorescent screen for pyruvate kinase deficiency; pyruvate kinase enzyme activity assay; methemoglobin (Hi) concentration

Table 20. (continued)

Defect	Assays
Intracorpuscular: Hemoglobinopathies	
Thalassemias and sickle cell diseases	Blood film morphology: sickle cells, target cells (codocytes), microcytosis, hypochromia, anisocytosis; hemoglobin electrophoresis, HGB A_2 concentration, Kleihauer-Betke stain
Intracorpuscular: Complement sensitivity	
Paroxysmal nocturnal hemoglobinemia (PNH)	Sugar water test, Ham acidified serum (obsolete), flow cytometry for RBC membrane complement regulatory proteins CD55 and CD59
Intracorpuscular: Acquired membrane disorders	
Vitamin E deficiency; abetalipoproteinemia; liver or renal failures	Blood film morphology: abnormal RBCs such as acanthocytes, macro-ovalocytes, and target cells (codocytes)
Extracorpuscular: Infections	
Intracellular: malaria, babesiosis *Extracellular:* bartonellosis, *Clostridium perfringens,* meningococcal or pneumococcal sepsis, viral infections	Blood film morphology for presence of organisms: thin and thick smears Blood and other body fluid cultures

Defect	Assays

Extracorpuscular: Mechanical

Macroangiopathic: heart valve, march hemoglobinuria	Complete blood cell count, peripheral blood film for
Microangiopathic: DIC, TTP, HUS, malignant hypertension	schistocytes, D-dimer level, prothrombin time (PT), partial thromboplastin time (PTT), fibrinogen, VWF-cleaving protease (ADAMTS-13) activity and inhibitor

Extracorpuscular: Chemicals and physical agents

Oxidative agents: high dose dapsone	Glucose-6-phosphate dehydrogenase, glutathione reductase or methemoglobin reductase enzyme activity
Non-oxidative agents: lead and venoms	Review of peripheral blood film for basophilic stippling in lead and other heavy metal poisoning
Osmotic effect: water (drowning or water irrigation in surgery); burns	Review of peripheral blood film for echinocytes (crenated cells, burr cells), stomatocytes

Extravascular Hemolysis

Extravascular hemolysis typically occurs in *warm autoimmune hemolytic anemia* (WAIHA), caused by IgG autoantibodies directed at RBC membrane antigens. Hemolysis is mediated by Fc receptor-bearing macrophages that phagocytize RBCs within the spleen and liver. A membrane fragment bearing the patchy antibody is removed, leaving the remaining membrane and its intracellular contents to reanneal and return to the circulation.

The peripheral blood morphologic hallmark is the *microspherocyte*, reflected in an elevated MCHC. Microspherocytes do not deform to traverse small vessels, are trapped, and have a shortened lifespan. This mediates chronic intravascular hemolysis to accompany the extravascular component. Microspherocytes are osmotically fragile as their membranes are inflexible and may be detected using the time-honored osmotic fragility test.

The *direct antiglobulin test* (DAT, direct Coombs) definitively differentiates immune from non-immune hemolytic anemias. The DAT is positive when IgG or complement component C3 is bound to the RBC membrane. A negative DAT in the presence of hemolysis leads to investigation of one of the non-immune causes listed in Table 20.

G6PD Deficiency Tests

Glucose-6-phosphate dehydrogenase (G6PD) is a red cell enzyme that protects the cell from oxidation damage. Although total deficiency of G6PD is probably incompatible with life, approximately 60 mutations or combinations of mutations have been documented in patients with varying degrees of enzyme deficiency. This deficiency is the most common metabolic disorder of erythrocytes, affecting up to 12% of African-American males. The patient suspected of being G6PD deficient should be initially screened with a rapid fluorescent spot test using EDTA anticoagulated blood. The assay is based on the generation of NADPH from NADP in the presence of G6PD. Lack of fluorescence is seen only in severely deficient cells, as the assay is insensitive to milder forms of G6PD deficiency. Furthermore, a false negative result occurs in marked reticulocytosis following a hemolytic episode, as reticulocytes have high enzyme activity. The screen is followed by a quantitative colorimetric assay when desired; however, reticulocytosis also falsely raises the quantitative result. A recently developed test based on allele-specific polymerase chain reaction (AS-PCR) is accurate and independent of the reticulocyte count. PCR tests detect specific mutations and can be used for population screening, family studies, or prenatal diagnosis.

PNH Diagnosis

Paroxysmal nocturnal hemoglobinuria (PNH) is an acquired stem cell mutation that leads to the proliferation of red cells, leukocytes, and platelets that lack a number of membrane proteins uniquely anchored by glycosylphosphatidylinositol (GPI). Among GPI-linked proteins are the decay accelerating factor (DAF or CD55) and membrane inhibitor of reactive lysis (MIRL or CD59), both proteins that protect red cells from complement lysis. In PNH, their absence explains the cell's increased sensitivity to hemolysis. The current diagnosis of PNH uses flow cytometry to document the absence of CD55 and CD59 from the red cell membrane. A more sensitive method replaces RBCs with neutrophils to detect the presence of these and other GPI-linked proteins. Neutrophils have normal survival time, while PNH red cells do not. Flow cytometry has virtually replaced the time-honored but cumbersome Ham test, as it is more sensitive and specific. Furthermore, flow quantitates the percentage of affected cells and aids in monitoring therapy.

Autoimmune Hemolytic Anemia (AIHA, 19,20)

Warm autoimmune hemolytic anemia (WAIHA) is the most common immune hemolytic anemia. An IgG autoantibody of vague specificity is directed at a common RBC membrane antigen. IgG antibodies bind RBC membranes most avidly at 37 °C, in contrast to IgM isotype "cold" agglutinins whose optimum temperature may be 4–6 °C Since IgG antibodies activate complement only when two molecules are in close proximity, most WAIHA cases fix no C3. Most hemolysis is extravascular, producing visible microspherocytes. Chronic lymphocytic leukemia (CLL), lymphoma, and autoimmune diseases such as systemic lupus erythematosus (SLE) are associated with WAIHA.

A specific AIHA subgroup is induced by penicillins, cephalosporins, and other drugs. History is the most efficient means to diagnose drug-induced AIHA, important because the condition may be fatal if the drug is not withdrawn (21).

Cold AIHA, usually called cold agglutinin disease (CAD), is mediated by an IgM autoantibody. Many cold agglutinins are asymptomatic, causing room temperature RBC agglutination in hematology laboratory specimens without clinical significance. Cold agglutinins with higher thermal ranges may cause pain, swelling, and blanching in extremities, known as Raynaud phenomenon, and occasional complement-mediated RBC lysis.

In patients with CAD, the DAT is positive for C3 because a single pentameric IgM molecule may activate complement. When present, hemolysis is predominantly intravascular. CAD may be primary or secondary, acute or chronic. In children, an acute transient episode of CAD may follow infection with Epstein-Barr virus; in adults, a similar presentation may complicate *Mycoplasma pneumoniae* infection. Lymphoproliferative conditions may cause chronic CAD with an episodic pattern of hemolysis alternating with stable phases.

Osmotic Fragility Test

The normal RBC membrane allows water to pass through while generally restricting solutes. Osmosis is the process by which cells shrink due to loss of water when placed in *hypertonic* solutions. Endosmosis is the absorption of water when the cells are in a *hypotonic* medium, which results in swelling and, ultimately, hemolysis. The osmotic fragility test determines the fragility of the RBC membrane by assessing the hemolytic effect of saline solutions of varying concentrations (Figure 15). The curve is used to interpret the osmotic fragility of the RBCs being tested. A patient sample should always be tested in parallel with a normal (control) sample. Incubation of the blood sample overnight at 37 °C increases the sensitivity of the test for increased osmotic fragility, and is done in most clinical laboratories. The shape and the position of the curve relative to the normal control provide information about the sample being evaluated. The concentration of NaCl solution causing 50% lysis is called the *median corpuscular fragility* (MCF; reference range: 0.40–0.45 g/dL). Furthermore, the concentration at which lysis begins (minimum resistance) and that at which lysis appears to be complete (maximum resistance) should also be calculated.

In HS due to lack of the cytoskeletal protein spectrin, the unstable membrane forces the cell to resemble a sphere, which characteristically increases the osmotic fragility. When testing these RBCs, their curve "shifts to the right" of the normal control RBCs (Figure 15). On the other hand, cells from patients with hemoglobinopathies such as sickle cell disease have decreased osmotic fragility. The latter occurs because HGB S is poorly soluble in low oxygen tension situations; it forms a gel and polymerizes into fibrilary structures or "tactoids" that distort the RBCs, causing them to become rigid and sickled. Thus, the curve obtained for a patient with sickle cell disease is expected to be "shifted to the left" (not shown). However, the osmotic fragility test should not be the only test used in the diagnosis of this condition, and sickle cell solubility test followed by hemoglobin electrophoresis should be done if clinically indicated. Furthermore, decreased osmotic fragility may be an artifact of the assay, such as during a rise in pH of the blood sample. If in doubt, repeat the assay (to ensure that experimental errors did not affect the results significantly) before diagnosing sickle cell anemia, some thalassemias, or any condition associated with decreased osmotic fragility.

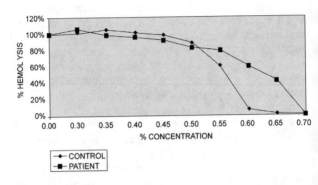

Figure 15. Osmotic fragility test. For the normal control, indicated by diamonds (reading right to left), hemolysis is slightly detectable in the 0.60% saline solution, reaches 60% in the 0.55% tube, and 100% in the 0.45% tube. The sample with HS (squares) exhibits 40% hemolysis at 0.65% saline concentration, and approaches complete hemolysis at 0.50%.

WBC Disorders

Table 21. Distributive and Morphologic WBC Changes

Condition	Morphology	Associations
Leukopenia	WBC count <3000/μL with normal morphology	Chemotherapy, idiosyncratic drug reactions, hematologic disease
Neutropenia	PMN counts <1500/μL with BANDs and immature forms in peripheral blood (left shift); may be accompanied by relative lymphocytosis, LYMPHs >3440/μL	Myeloid suppression, immunosuppression, splenic sequestration, chemotherapy, idiosyncratic drug reactions, margination of circulating PMN pool, or peripheral consumption as in infection
Leukocytosis	WBC count >11,000/μL: PMNs >8030/μL, BANDs >1210/μL (left shift), toxic granules, cytoplasmic vacuoles and Döhle bodies; or LYMPH count >3440/μL with variant LYMPHs	Inflammation, infection, hematologic disease, post-chemotherapy marrow recovery
Neutrophilia Neutrophilic Leukocytosis	PMN count >8030/μL with BANDs >1210/μL and immature forms in peripheral blood (left shift), toxic granulation, cytoplasmic vacuoles, and Döhle bodies	Inflammation, infection, hematologic disease, post-chemotherapy marrow recovery

Continued

Table 21. (continued)

Condition	Morphology	Associations
Eosinophilia	EO count >400/μL with band forms and, rarely, eosinophilic myelocytes	Allergic disorders, parasitic infestation, drug reaction, collagen vascular diseases, and malignancies such as Hodgkin lymphoma
Basophilia	BASO count >220/μL with rare immature forms	Myeloproliferative disorders, especially CML
Monocytosis	MONO count >1430/μL with rare immature forms	Chronic infections, collagen vascular diseases, and post-chemotherapy marrow recovery
Lymphocytosis	Mature small LYMPH count >3440/μL with a few large variants (activated, atypical, reactive LYMPHs)	Chronic immunologic stimulation, viral infections like Epstein-Barr virus (EBV). In post-chemotherapy state, lymphocytosis is relative
Leukemoid reaction	Severe neutrophilia with BANDs and early immature myeloid stages	Reactive process, certain bacterial infections
Leukoerythroblastic picture	Severe neutrophilia with BANDs and early immature myeloid stages plus nucleated RBCs	Myelophthisic conditions such as myelofibrosis, metastatic tumors, leukemia, and granulomas. Severe hemolysis and massive blood loss

Table 22. WBC, RBC, and Platelet Artifacts

Artifact	Morphology	Associations
WBC fragmentation	Fragments of PMNs or LYMPHs	Storage in EDTA longer than 24 hours
Cytoplasmic vacuoles	Non-staining cytoplasmic areas in PMNs, LYMPHs and MONOs	Toxic changes, infection, and EDTA storage longer than 24 hours
Smudge cells	Ballooning of nuclei and loss of cytoplasm	Lymphocytosis >4330/µL associated with chronic lymphocytic leukemia (CLL) and in some acute lymphoblastic leukemias (ALLs)
RBC agglutination (clumping)	Macroscopically visible irregular, coarse RBC agglutination	Cold hemagglutinin, also called cold agglutinin disease
Rouleaux	Linear RBC stacking	Paraproteinemias (myeloma) and other dysproteinemias
Platelet clumping	Platelet clumps in thin part of blood film and at feather edge	Partial clotting when EDTA tube is not mixed; EDTA-related clumping associated with satellitism
Platelet satellitism (satellitosis)	Platelet adhesion to WBCs, usually PMNs	Exposure of neoantigen in EDTA tube, no clinical consequence except for false thrombocytopenia

Table 23. WBC Distribution and Kinetics

Cell lineage	Distribution	Growth Factors
PMNs: SEGs and BANDs	Maturation in bone marrow and release into peripheral blood. PMNs alternate between circulating and marginating pool. Marginating PMNs roll, tether, attach to endothelium, and extravasate (exit) into tissues	G-CSF and GM-CSF
EOs	Circulating and marginating pools	GM-CSF, IL-3 and IL-5
BASOs and mast cells	Rare in blood, abundant in tissue	GM-CSF, IL-3, IL-5; c-kit ligand specific to mast cells
MONOs	Circulating and marginating pools, <8 hours in peripheral blood	GM-CSF
LYMPHs	B cells circulate several days or months and T cells circulate for several years	Antigen exposure, IL-2 and IL-3

Myeloproliferative Disorders (MPD, 22,23)

Chronic Myelogenous Leukemia (CML)

CML is the most common MPD. It typically presents with an elevated WBC and platelet count and basophilia.

CML Morphology

Peripheral blood: Sustained leukocytosis >20,000/µL; thrombocytosis >400,000/µL; basophilia >220/µL; neutrophil alkaline phosphatase (NAP, leukocyte alkaline phosphatase, LAP) score <10, blasts <5%. In accelerated phase the NAP is variable.

Bone marrow: Hypercellular marrow (>80%) with early and late myeloid cells called "myelocyte bulge," blasts <5%, and small megakaryocytes. Myelofibrosis appears in accelerated phase.

CML Diagnosis

- Karyotyping, reverse transcriptase PCR, and FISH; Philadelphia chromosome t(9:22)(q34;q11)
- BCR-ABL fusion:
  - m-BCR p190 (e1a1) associated with acute lymphoblastic leukemia (ALL)
  - M-BCR p210 (e13a2 or e14a2) found in typical CML
  - µ-BCR p230 (e19a2) seen in indolent CML such as chronic neutrophilia and thrombocytosis

CML Blast Crisis

Leukocytosis with blasts ≥20%; myeloblasts in 60–70% of cases, lymphoblasts in 25–30%, multilineage blasts in 10–15%.

Polycythemia Vera (PV)

PV is a clonal proliferation of erythroid, megakaryocytic, and myeloid elements in bone marrow with an increased RBC count, HGB, HCT, and RBC mass. There are no gross chromosomal defects. The JAK-2 mutation is found in approximately 50% of cases. In PV, erythroid progenitors grow independently of erythropoietin and exhibit increased sensitivity to interleukin-3, GM-CSF, and stem cell factor.

PV Morphology

Peripheral blood: Elevated RBC count, HGB, HCT, WBC, and platelet counts.

Bone marrow: Hypercellular marrow, trilineage hyperplasia, giant megakaryocytes with clustering; increased reticulin (late stage); *absent iron stores* as a result of therapeutic phlebotomy.

PV Differential Diagnosis

- Relative erythrocytosis in stress, spurious polycythemia, or Gaisbock syndrome
- Smokers' polycythemia
- Secondary polycythemia in lung disease, erythropoietin-producing tumors
- Essential thrombocythemia

Essential Thrombocythemia (ET)

ET is a sustained thrombocytosis >700,000 platelets/μL with no other CBC abnormalities and no gross chromosomal defects.

ET Morphology

Peripheral blood: Thrombocytosis, mild or no leukocytosis, and normal HGB.

Bone marrow, early phase: Megakaryocyte clustering, increased ploidy and size; slight increase of fine reticulin; uninvolved intervening marrow with normal erythroid and myeloid elements.

Bone marrow, late phase: Megakaryocyte clustering with increased ploidy and size; marrow fibrosis with marked increase of reticulin.

ET Differential Diagnosis

Differentiate from thrombocytosis secondary to inflammation, malignancy, or hemorrhage; other MPDs.

ET Diagnosis

ET is a sustained thrombocytosis of >700,000/μL. JAK-2 mutation is present in 30–50% of patients. Erythroblastic progenitors show increased sensitivity to erythropoietin and megakaryocytes to thrombopoietin.

Chronic Idiopathic (or Agnogenic) Myelofibrosis with Myeloid Metaplasia (MMM, AMMM)

MMM is extramedullary hematopoiesis secondary to reactive myelofibrosis; considered to be a stem cell disorder of unknown etiology and no demonstrable chromosomal abnormalities.

MMM Morphology

Peripheral blood: Anemia in 50%; leukocytosis in 40%; thrombocytopenia in 25%; leukopenia in 20%; thrombocytosis in 20%; leuko-erythroblastic picture, poikilocytosis, and dacryocytes (teardrop RBCs) in 100%.

Bone marrow: Marrow is hypercellular during cellular phase. There is reticulin fibrosis in early or late phase.

Spleen: Massive splenomegaly >2 kg with extramedullary hematopoiesis.

MMM Differential Diagnosis

Differentiate from acute leukemia; acute myelosclerosis; acute megakaryocytic leukemia (M7); hairy cell leukemia; metastatic carcinoma; non-Hodgkin or Hodgkin lymphoma; myelodysplastic syndrome; multiple myeloma with polyneuropathy, organomegaly, endocrinopathy, monoclonal "M" protein and skin manifestations (POEMS).

Myelodysplastic Syndromes (MDS)

Definition: The myelodysplastic syndromes (MDSs) are a heterogeneous group of hematologic disorders with peripheral *cytopenia* and *hypercellular marrow,* increase of *blasts,* and *dyshematopoiesis* (dysplasia). MDS is more frequently diagnosed in the elderly and both primary and secondary MDS is on the rise. A recent study estimates 8.6% incidence of treatment-related MDS (TMDS, 23); another reports 12% incidence in patients who received high-dose chemotherapy followed by bone marrow transplantation for Hodgkin and non-Hodgkin lymphoma (24).

Traditional classification systems (FAB and REAL/WHO) are based on peripheral blood and bone marrow aspirate smear findings. Bone marrow biopsy findings are not included in any classification scheme. Clinical outcomes depend on severity of cytopenias, bone marrow blasts, and abnormal karyotype. See the international prognostic scoring system (IPSS) below.

Common Laboratory Findings for Most MDS Types (25,26)

Blood

- Macrocytosis
- Leukopenia
- Neutrophil hyposegmentation and hypogranulation (pseudo Pelger-Huet cells)
- Monocytosis in chronic myelomonocytic leukemia (CMML)
- Immature myeloid cells
- Normal or decreased platelet count

Bone Marrow

- Hypercellular marrow in the majority of MDS patients
- Dyserythropoiesis with megaloblastic changes and ringed sideroblasts, especially in refractory anemia with ringed sideroblasts (RARS)
- Increase of early myeloid cells and blasts with dysplastic features
- Micro-megakaryocytes in 5q- syndrome
- Altered marrow topography with early fibrosis

MDS: Differential Diagnosis

- Megaloblastic anemia caused by B_{12} or folate deficiency
- Myeloproliferative disorders: CML, PV, ET
- Congenital dyserythropoietic anemia (CDA)
- Heavy metal poisoning such as arsenic
- Drug effects caused by chemotherapy and antibiotics
- HIV infection
- Chronic infections that may cause monocytosis
- Marrow suppression: must exclude aplastic anemia
- Secondary myelodysplastic syndromes
- Marrow fibrosis and tumor infiltration

Table 24. 2002 MDS Classification by World Health Organization (WHO)

Myelodysplastic Syndromes	Peripheral Blood	Bone Marrow
Refractory anemia (RA)	Anemia None or rare blasts Monocytes 1,430–10,000/μL	Erythroid dysplasia only <10% dysplastic myelocytes or megakaryocytes <5% blasts <15% ringed sideroblasts
Refractory anemia with ringed sideroblasts (RARS)	Anemia Dimorphic RBC population No blasts	Erythroid dysplasia <10% dysplastic myelocytes or megakaryocytes ≥15% ringed sideroblasts <5% blasts
Refractory cytopenia with multi-lineage dysplasia (RCMD)	Cytopenias in two cell lineages or pancytopenia Monocytes 1,430–10,000/μL None or rare blasts No Auer rods	Dysplasia in ≥10% of cells in two or more myeloid cell lineages <5% blasts No Auer rods <15% ringed sideroblasts
Refractory cytopenia with multi-lineage dysplasia with ringed sideroblasts (RCMD-RS)	Cytopenias in two cell lineages or pancytopenia Monocytes 1,430–10,000/μL No Auer rods	Dysplasia in ≥10% of cells in two or more myeloid cell lineages <5% blasts No Auer rods

	Blood	Bone Marrow
	None or rare blasts	>15% ringed sideroblasts
Refractory anemia with excess blasts (RAEB-1)	Cytopenias <5% blasts No Auer rods Monocytes 1430–10,000/µL	One or multilineage dysplasia Hypercellular marrow (rarely hypoplastic) 5–9% blasts No Auer rods
Refractory anemia with excess blasts (RAEB-2)	Cytopenias 5–19% blasts ± Auer rods Monocytes 1430–10,000/µL	One or multilineage dysplasia Hypercellular marrow (rarely hypoplastic) 5–19% blasts ± Auer rods
MDS-unclassified	Cytopenias No or rare blasts No Auer rods	Unilineage myeloid or megakaryocytic dysplasia <5% blasts No Auer rods
Myelodysplastic syndrome associated with isolated del (5q)	Macrocytic anemia <5% blasts Normal platelet count or >400,000/µL	Normal to increased megakaryocytes with hypolobated nuclei <5% blasts No Auer rods Isolated del (5q)

Continued

Table 24. (continued)

Myelodysplastic/ Myeloproliferative Disorders	Peripheral Blood	Bone Marrow
Chronic myelomonocytic leukemia (CMML)	Leukocytosis and monocytosis Anemia, variable platelet counts	Packed marrow with all three cell lineages and increase of monocytes
Atypical chronic myelogenous leukemia	Leukocytosis with atypical myeloid forms	Packed marrow with myeloid predominance
Juvenile myelomonocytic	Leukocytosis, myeloid left-shift and	Packed marrow and immature

Table 25. International Prognostic Scoring System (IPSS) for MDS (27)

Parameter	Criteria	Score
Blast count in BM	<5%	0.0
	5–10%	0.5
	11–20%	1.5
	21–30%	2.0
Karyotype	Normal or 5q-	0.0
	Other	0.5
	Three abnormalities or complex karyotype	1.0
Cytopenias	None or one lineage	0.0
	Two or three lineages	0.5

- Low (score of 0) = median survival of 5.7 years
- Intermediate (0.5 or 1.0) = median survival of 3.5 years
- Intermediate (1.5 or 2.0) = median survival of 1.2 years
- High (>2.5) = median survival of 0.4 years

MPD / MDS / Final Outcome

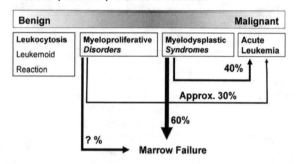

Figure 16. Association of MPDs, MDSs, and acute leukemia.
Spectrum of bone marrow abnormalities with the expected percentage of cases that will convert to marrow failure or acute leukemia.

Acute Leukemia

Acute leukemia is defined by increased blasts, the most immature identifiable form of myeloid and lymphoid cell lineages, to >20% in the bone marrow and blood. Blasts may infiltrate other tissues. Absolute blast counts in the peripheral blood range from <1000/μL to >100,000/μL. Marrow is typically hypercellular, but occasionally may be hypocellular. Hypocellular marrow is called *aleukemic* leukemia or *hypoplastic* leukemia.

Clinical Features of Acute Leukemia

Pallor and lethargy due to anemia, chronic and recurrent infections due to neutropenia, spontaneous bruises due to thrombocytopenia, fever, anorexia, and malaise. Disseminated intravascular coagulation (DIC) is seen in M3 due to the release of procoagulant granules from the neoplastic promyelocytes. Leukemic organ infiltration causes tender bones in children, lymphadenopathy and meningeal syndrome in acute lymphoblastic leukemia (ALL), gum hypertrophy and bleeding in acute myelomonocytic and acute monocytic leukemia (FAB classifications M4 and M5), skin involvement, and ovarian and testicular swelling.

Acute Leukemia Classification (28)

The acute leukemias are classified using the French American British (FAB, 1976) scheme based on Wright-Giemsa cell morphology and cytochemistry in blood and bone marrow, or using the World Health Organization (WHO, 2001) scheme based on Wright-Giemsa morphology, cytochemistry, immunochemistry markers, phenotyping, mutations, and transformation from pre-existing conditions.

Table 26. Acute Leukemia Risk Factors

Heredity	Down and Bloom syndrome: 20- to 30-fold increase of AML
Oncogene activation	t(15;17): in acute promyelocytic leukemia (APL, M3), fusion of truncated retinoic acid receptor (RARAα) on chromosome 17 with PML gene on chromosome 15
	t(9;22): in chronic myelogenous leukemia (CML), fusion of BCR on chromosome 22 with ABL on chromosome 9 yielding 9q+ ABL/BCR and 22q–
	MYC in Burkitt lymphoma t(8;14)
	Bcl-2 in other lymphomas
Toxic exposure	Benzene
Other risk factors	Ionizing radiation, infection with human T lymphotrophic virus 1 (HTLV-1), or Epstein-Barr virus (EBV)
	Myelodysplastic syndromes and myeloproliferative disorders
	Secondary leukemias: post-chemotherapy or radiation therapy (rapidly growing group)

Laboratory Diagnosis of Acute Leukemia

Peripheral Blood Films and Data from Analyzers

- Blast flag from analyzer
- Blasts >20% and other immature myeloid or lymphoid cells in blood film examination
- Markedly elevated or decreased WBC count
- Normocytic/normochromic anemia with reduced HGB, HCT, and RBC count
- Marked thrombocytopenia

Bone Marrow Biopsy and Aspirate

- Morphology: >20% blasts, dyspoiesis, dysplasia
- Abnormal localization of precursors (ALIP)
- Hypercellularity

Cytochemistry

Myeloperoxidase (MPO), Sudan black B (SBB), non-specific (NSE) and specific esterases, periodic acid Schiff (PAS), tartrate-resistant acid phosphatase (TRAP), neutrophil alkaline phosphatase (NAP or leukocyte alkaline phosphatase, LAP)

Immunologic Markers by Flow Cytometry (Refer to Flow Cytometry)

- B lineage markers: CD19, 20, 21; cytoplasmic (cIg) and surface immunoglobulin (sIg)
- T lineage markers: CD2, 3, 4, 5, 7, 8
- NK lineage markers: CD3 surface-negative, CD16, 56, 57
- Myeloid markers: CD11, 13, 15, 33, 34
- Megakaryocytic lineage markers: CD41, 61; factor VIII antigen

Cytogenetics (Karyotyping):

Translocations, inversions, deletions

Molecular Diagnosis

Refer to fluorescent in-situ hybridization, FISH; polymerase chain reaction, PCR

Table 27. Acute Leukemias with Recurrent Chromosomal Defects (WHO Classification) (29)

Category	Cell Morphology	Cell Surface Markers	Cytogenetics	Prognosis
Acute myeloblastic anemia (AML) with t(8;21)	Large blasts with basophilic cytoplasm, abnormal granules, Auer rods, dysplasia, maturing myeloid cells	CD13, 19, 33, 34, 117	t(8;21)(q22;q22) *AML1/ETO*	More favorable than AML without recurrent genetic abnormalities
AML with inv(16)	Myelomonocytic blasts, increased immature eosinophils, biphasic granules (eosinophilic/basophilic	CD4, 13, 14, 33, 64	Inv(16)(p13;q22) or t(16;16)(p13;q22)	More favorable than other AMLs
Acute promyelocytic leukemia t(15;17)	Promyelocytes with bright azurophilic granules, Auer rods, hypogranular variants	CD2±, 13, 33, 64±; HLA-DR negative	t(15;17)(q22;q12) *PML/RARα* variants all involve 17q12	Good prognosis when responsive to all-trans retinoic acid (ATRA)
AML with 11q23	Variable. Monocytic differentiation seen with t(9;11)	CD4, 13, 14, 33, 34, 56±, 57 CD36 with monocytic differentiation	t(9;11)(p22;q23), others	Poor prognosis

				Median survival <3 years
AML, therapy-related	Multilineage dysplasia, ringed sideroblasts, increased basophils	CD13, 33, 34, 56±, 57	11q23 abnormality seen with topoisomerase II inhibitor-associated AML	

CD: cluster of differentiation; Inv: inversion; t: translocation

Table 28. Acute Myeloblastic Leukemias, Not Otherwise Categorized (WHO and FAB Classification)

Category	Cell Morphology	Cell Surface Markers	Cytogenetics	Prognosis
AML, minimally differentiated (M0)	Blasts with minimal differentiation, no cytoplasmic granules	CD33dim, 34, 117; TdT±	No consistent cytogenetic abnormality	Variable
AML without maturation (M1)	Mostly myeloblasts and no maturation, rare Auer rods	CD13, 15, 33, 34, 117	No consistent cytogenetic abnormality	Variable
Acute myelomonocytic leukemia (M4)	Myeloid blasts (~20–80%) and monoblasts	CD13, 14, 15 bright, 33, 64	No consistent cytogenetic abnormality	Variable

Continued

Table 28. (continued)

Category	Cell Morphology	Cell Surface Markers	Cytogenetics	Prognosis
Acute monocytic (M5) a, b	>80% monoblasts	CD14, 15 bright, 33, 64	No consistent cytogenetic abnormality	Poor when there is early visceral involvement
Acute erythroleukemia (M6) a, b	Cytoplasmic vacuoles in erythroid blasts, dyserythropoiesis, few myeloid blasts M6a is pure erythroid leukemia	CD13, 33, 71, 117; erythroid: glycophorin, PAS stain +	Multiple chromosome defects	Poor, bone marrow failure
Acute megakaryoblastic leukemia (M7)	Blasts with cytoplasmic projections and marrow fibrosis	CD33, 41, 61	No consistent cytogenetic abnormality	Variable
Acute basophilic leukemia	Basophilic granules in the blasts	CD13, 15, 33	No consistent cytogenetic abnormality	Variable

CD: cluster of differentiation; TdT: terminal deoxynucleotidyl transferase

Table 29. Acute Lymphoblastic Leukemia

Category	Cell Morphology	Cell Surface Markers	Cytogenetics	Prognosis
Precursor B	Small to large blasts with minimal cytoplasm	CD10, 19, 34; TdT+	t(12;21) (p12;q22), t(9;22), 11q23, t(4;11) (q21;q23)	Better than AML
Precursor T	Small to large blasts with variable cytoplasm	CD1a, 2, 3, 4/8, 10±; TdT±	No specific abnormality	Variable

CD: cluster of differentiation; TdT: terminal deoxynucleotidyl transferase; t: translocation

Table 30. Acute Leukemia, Therapy-Related

Category	Cell Morphology	Cell Surface Markers	Cytogenetics	Prognosis
Alkylating agent	Blasts, multilineage dysplasia, increased ringed sideroblasts	CD13, 33, 34, 56±, 57	Multiple	Variable, poor
Topoisomerase	Blasts, multilineage dysplasia, increased ringed sideroblasts	CD13, 33, 34, 56±, 57	11q23	Poor, <3 yr

Table 31. Acute Leukemia of Ambiguous or Biphenotypic Lineage [Mixed features and markers of myeloid and lymphoid lineages; classify by European group for the immunological classification of leukemia (EGIL) scoring system]

Score	B-lymphoid	T-lymphoid	Myeloid
2	Cytoplasmic CD22	Membrane/	Myeloperoxidase
	Cytoplasmic CD79a	cytoplasmic CD3	
	Cytoplasmic IgM	Anti-T-LYMPH	
		receptor	
1	CD10	CD2	CD13
	CD19	CD5	CD33
	CD20	CD8	CD65
		CD10	CD117
0.5	CD24	CD1a	CD14
	TdT	CD7	CD15
		TdT	CD64

Myeloid lineage, AML-M0: myeloid score ≥4, lymphoid score ≤3
Lymphoid lineage, T or B: lymphoid score ≥4, myeloid score ≤3
Bi-phenotypic lineage: T or B lymphoid and myeloid score each ≥2 and ≤4

Table 32. Acute Leukemia Prognosis: Treatment Response Predictors

Factor	Good	Poor
AML		++
ALL in children	++++	
WBC count	Reduced	Elevated
Immunophenotype	CD10+	AML and B-ALL
Age	Child 2–12 years old	Adult or child <2 years old
Cytogenetics	Normal or hyperdiploidy	Philadelphia chromosome and other translocations
Time to remission	<4 weeks	>4 weeks
CNS disease	Absent	Present
Mixed lineage		++++

Lymphocytic Disorders

Chronic Lymphocytic Leukemia (CLL)

CLL is the most common leukemia in adults over 60 years old, and represents approximately 30% of all leukemias (NIH data, 2005). CLL presents as asymptomatic peripheral lymphocytosis with nodal enlargement followed by marrow involvement.

CLL morphology: The majority of WBCs in the blood and bone marrow are small, mature-appearing lymphoid cells with dense chromatin. Less than 20% prolymphocytes may be present. In transformation to prolymphocytic leukemia (PLL), >55% are prolymphocytes, large lymphoid cells with prominent central nucleoli. PLL usually has WBC counts > 80,000/μL.

In small cell lymphoma (SLL) the primary presentation is in tissue without marrow or peripheral blood involvement; however, the neoplastic cells in SLL are identical to those in CLL. Lymph nodes and other hematopoietic tissues are effaced by diffuse infiltration composed mostly of small lymphoid cells interspersed among a few large cells, forming "pseudo-growth centers." These activated lymphocytes and prolymphocytes begin as a small part of the infiltrate; however, they become more frequent in prolymphocytic large cell transformation.

CLL Immunophenotype

- CLL/SLL: CD20+(dim); CD19+; CD5+; CD23+; dim κ or λ light chains
- PLL: CD19+; CD20+(bright); CD5+/−; bright κ or λ light chains; κ FMC-7+; CD25+

CLL Differential Diagnosis

- Mantle cell lymphoma in leukemic phase
- Marginal zone lymphoma; extranodal, nodal, and splenic form
- PLL needs to be differentiated from lymphoma

CLL Prognosis

CLL and SLL are indolent conditions with median survival of more than 12 years after initial diagnosis. Morphology is a poor predictor of outcomes and survival depends on the factors in Table 33.

Table 33. CLL Prognosis

Factor	Prognosis	Factor	Prognosis
Normal karyotype	Favorable	ZAP 70+ >20% (30)	Poor
13q del	Favorable	High β2-microglobulin	Poor
Mutated IgVH	Favorable	Unmutated IgVH	Poor
Low levels of IL-6	Favorable	11q del	Poor
Trisomy	Intermediate	17p del	Very poor
CD38+ >30%	Poor	Diffuse bone marrow involvement	Poor

IgVH: Immunoglobulin variable region.

Other Lymphoproliferative Conditions and Leukemias

Table 34 delineates low- to high-grade lymphoproliferative conditions characterized by peripheral blood lymphocytosis with tissue and organ infiltration. The classification is based on immunophenotype (T, B LYMPH or NK cell type) and morphology.

Table 34. Other Lymphoproliferative Disorders by Morphology, Phenotype, and Molecular Diagnosis

Condition	Morphology	Cell Surface Markers and Diagnosis	Molecular Findings and Prognosis
Hairy cell leukemia (HCL)	Variable LYMPH diameter, gray cytoplasm, some with hairy projections. Large reticulated nucleus. Marrow reticulin fibrosis causes dry tap with no marrow aspirate	CD11c, 19, 20, 25, 103 and κ or λ light chain restriction; TRAP+	No specific molecular or cytogenetic abnormalities. Indolent disease and long remission after treatment
Large granular lymphocytic leukemia (LGL) or proliferation	Peripheral blood LYMPHs with abundant cytoplasm containing azurophilic granules and nuclei with condensed chromatin. Bone marrow may be negative	CD2, 3, 16, 56±, 57; positive TRC-γ gene rearrangements	No specific molecular or cytogenetic abnormalities. Indolent condition and long remission after treatments

Continued

85

Table 34. (continued)

Condition	Morphology	Cell Surface Markers and Diagnosis	Molecular Findings and Prognosis
Natural killer (NK) cell leukemia	Variable LYMPH diameter, gray-blue cytoplasm with granules	CD2, 56, 57; CD3 negative	Aggressive disease with short survival
Adult T-cell leukemia/lymphoma (ATLL)	Marked leukocytosis, variable LYMPH diameter with nuclear irregularities (clover-leaf) Bone marrow usually packed with leukemic cells	CD2, 3, 4, 25; positive TCR-γ and HTLV1	No specific molecular or cytogenetic abnormalities Aggressive disease with short survival
T-prolymphocytic leukemia	Variable LYMPH diameter, some with irregular nuclear outline	CD2, 3, 4 or 7 (variable) and TCR+	Indolent to aggressive
T-γ/δ leukemia	Small- to medium-sized lymphoid cells	CD2, 3, 4, 8 (negative)	Indolent to aggressive

Plasma Cell Proliferative Disorders

A group of disorders characterized by proliferation of plasma cells and plasmacytoid lymphocytes with light chain or heavy chain restriction called a monoclonal gammopathy. Monoclonal protein (M-protein, para-protein) is produced by a clone of plasma cells and is made of one class of immunoglobulin heavy chain (γ, μ, α, δ, ε) and one type of light chain (κ or λ). The clinical spectrum ranges from benign or indolent to overtly malignant.

Classification of Plasma Cell Disorders

- Monoclonal gammopathy of undetermined significance (MGUS)
  - Benign, indolent condition with no specific etiology for monoclonal protein secretion. Approximately 20% develop into plasma cell myelomas (10- to 15-year follow-up by the Mayo Clinic).

- Malignant monoclonal gammopathies
  - Multiple myeloma; diffuse process, several sites
  - Plasmacytoma; solitary osseus or extraosseous location
  - Indolent myeloma; meets all criteria of myeloma without anemia
  - Waldenstrom macroglobulinemia
  - Heavy chain disease; Ig heavy chain fragments
  - Primary amyloidosis

Laboratory Methods

- Serum protein electrophoresis (SPEP) for detection of gammopathy
- Immunoelectrophoresis (IEP) and immunofixation (IF)
- Quantitative immunoglobulins by nephelometry
- 24-hour urine protein determination

Table 35. Frequency of Gammopathies

IgG	52%	Light chain only	11%
IgA	21%	Heavy chain only	1%
IgM	12%	Nonsecretory	1%
IgD	2%	Biclonal	<1%
IgE	<0.01%		

Major Diagnostic Criteria for Myeloma

Any two are needed for diagnosis:
- Bone marrow plasmacytosis >20% and/or plasma cell aggregates or clusters
- Extraosseous plasmacytoma
- Monoclonal gammopathy: IgG >35 g/L and IgA >20 g/L
- Urinary light chain excretion of >1g/24 hours

Minor Diagnostic Criteria

One or more together with one major criterion are needed for diagnosis:
- Marrow plasmacytosis <30%
- Lytic bone lesions
- Evidence of a monoclonal protein at lower concentration than above
- Hypoglobulinemia of normal proteins

Pathology and Molecular Cytogenetics

Bone marrow plasma cell infiltrates of >15% and paraprotein are usually present at the time of diagnosis. However, diagnosis depends on clinical disease: anemia secondary to marrow replacement, hypercalcemia, osteolytic lesions, paraprotein (M-protein) with suppression of normal immunoglobulin levels and marrow plasmacytosis. Cytogenetic analysis is difficult due to lack of mitosis in plasma cells; however, interphase FISH analysis may identify deletions of 13q14, 17p13, and 7q. Also, t(1;14)(q13;q32) may sometimes be present. Multiple drug resistance and poor prognosis is associated with 13q and 7q deletions.

Thrombocytopenia

Thrombocytopenia describes a platelet count less than 150,000/μL. However, since reference intervals represent the values of 95% of the healthy population, 2.5% of normal individuals are expected to have a platelet count below the reference range. While thrombocytopenia is the most common cause of bleeding, *spontaneous bleeding* is seen only when the platelet count drops below 50,000/μL. Further, the risk of spontaneous *life-threatening hemorrhage*, particularly into the central nervous system, rises significantly when the platelet count drops below 20,000/μL.

Thrombocytopenia and/or platelet dysfunction cause *mucocutaneous* bleeding, forming petechiae and bruising in the skin, and gingival bleeding, epistaxis, hematemesis, and menorrhagia from mucosal surfaces. When checking the history of a patient with thrombocytopenia, it is important to note current medications, past and current comorbidities, and social and family history for clues regarding the etiology of the abnormality. Microscopic review of platelet number and morphology during a peripheral blood film examination is essential. Thus, history and initial laboratory exams are crucial for proper patient management because treatments are etiology-specific and vary considerably.

Occasionally, patients will have *pseudo-thrombocytopenia*, a benign thrombocytopenia caused by platelet clumps or platelet satellitism (satellitosis) around neutrophils (31). A citrated blood sample with a blue closure often prevents satellitism and allows for an accurate platelet count.

There are three categories of thrombocytopenia: impaired marrow production, splenic sequestration, and accelerated destruction (Table 36).

Table 36. Mechanisms of Thrombocytopenia

Impaired production	Sequestration	Increased destruction
Alcohol	Cirrhosis with portal	Immune: ITP, drug-
Viral infections	hypertension	induced (HIT), PTP
Drugs	Splenomegaly in	Non-immune:
Vitamin deficiencies	leukemia or	DIC, TTP-HUS,
Bone marrow	lymphoma	malignant
metastases or		hypertension
fibrosis		

ITP: Immune thrombocytopenic purpura; HIT: heparin induced thrombocytopenia; PTP: post-transfusion purpura; DIC: disseminated intravascular coagulation; TTP/HUS: thrombotic thrombocytopenic purpura/hemolytic uremic syndrome

Impaired Marrow Platelet Production

Bone marrow examination readily establishes a platelet production defect by detecting fibrosis, tumor invasion, or a decreased number of megakaryocytes. In addition to megakaryocytes, bone marrow damage also affects normoblastic and myelocytic lineages, leading to varying degrees of anemia and leukopenia. Cytotoxic bone marrow injury occurs with alcohol or chemotherapeutic agents, directly affecting megakaryocyte proliferation and maturation. As many as 80% of hospitalized alcoholics have mild thrombocytopenia, though rarely below $100,000/\mu L$ (32). Since chronic alcoholism also leads to cirrhosis and splenic sequestration, more severe thrombocytopenia afflicts cirrhotic patients, often $65,000–75,000/\mu L$ (33).

Recovery from rubella, mumps, varicella, parvovirus, hepatitis C, and Epstein-Barr virus causes a transient, generally asymptomatic thrombocytopenia. HIV damages megakaryocytes, explaining why thrombocytopenia is a common finding in AIDS. Chemotherapeutic agents and radiation may cause permanent bone marrow fibrosis and long-term pancytopenia (34,35). Vitamin B_{12} and folate deficiencies may also cause thrombocytopenia, especially in persons who have intestinal disorders or pernicious anemia, or in the elderly. Congenital causes of thrombocytopenia such as Fanconi anemia and thrombocytopenia with absent radii (TAR) are rare and variable in their etiology and presentation (36).

Splenic Sequestration of Platelets

The spleen harbors approximately one-third of the total platelet mass. In massive splenomegaly, which may be detected on physical exam or by imaging studies, the spleen may sequester up to 90% of the body's platelet pool (37). Hypersplenism, defined as an increase in the activity of the reticuloendothelial system, often accompanies splenomegaly. Thrombocytopenia due to splenic sequestration alone rarely causes hemorrhage. In patients with more severe thrombocytopenia, a concomitant process such as immune thrombocytopenic purpura (ITP) should be excluded. If ITP is diagnosed, splenectomy may be indicated as a treatment strategy. In thrombocytopenia due to splenic sequestration, platelet transfusions are generally ineffective because the transfused platelets remain in the spleen.

Accelerated Destruction of Platelets

Several immune and non-immune causes of accelerated destruction are listed in Table 37.

Immune-Mediated Thrombocytopenia

Autoimmune diseases such as systemic lupus erythematosus, rheumatoid arthritis, and thyroiditis may be accompanied by variable thrombocytopenia; the degree of platelet decrease depends on compensatory increase of bone marrow megakaryocytes. A platelet-specific antibody assay may help identify the cause of the thrombocytopenia.

Table 37. Differential Diagnosis of Thrombocytopenia Caused by Accelerated Platelet Destruction

Condition	Associated Laboratory Findings
Immune thrombocytopenia	
ITP	Platelet-specific antibodies, large platelets, increased bone marrow megakaryocytes
Evans syndrome	Hemolytic anemia with microspherocytes; positive DAT; platelet antibodies
HIT	Antibodies to platelet factor 4
Non-immune thrombocytopenia	
DIC	D-dimers >10,000 ηg/mL; prolonged PT and PTT; hypofibrinogenemia*; MAHA; elevated LDH; hyperbilirubinemia; low or absent haptoglobin
TTP-HUS	MAHA; elevated LDH; hyperbilirubinemia; low or absent haptoglobin; D-dimers slightly elevated; variable BUN and creatinine

DIC: disseminated intravascular coagulation; PT: prothrombin time; PTT: partial thromboplastin time; LDH: lactate dehydrogenase; TTP: thrombotic thrombocytopenic purpura; HUS: hemolytic uremic syndrome; BUN: blood urea nitrogen; ITP: immune thrombocytopenic purpura; DAT: direct antiglobulin test; HIT: heparin-induced thrombocytopenia; MAHA: microangiopathic hemolytic anemia with schistocytes.
*Fibrinogen level may be normal despite increased consumption because it is an acute phase reactant.

ITP is a diagnosis of exclusion. Patients are generally asymptomatic except for mucocutaneous bleeding such as petechiae, bruising, epistaxis, or heavy menstrual periods. Because the accelerated bone marrow turnover releases an increased number of large platelets, patients are not generally at risk for severe organ or intracerebral hemorrhage despite severe thrombocytopenia.

Laboratory tests for ITP include direct platelet-bound and indirect serum antibody assays with follow-up antibody specificity tests. Except for the specificity assays, these are not sensitive or specific for ITP and not uniformly used.

Evans syndrome is characterized by ITP and autoimmune hemolytic anemia (AIHA) with severe thrombocytopenia and hemolysis.

Heparin-Induced Thrombocytopenia (HIT)

Among the many drugs that can cause thrombocytopenia, heparin is probably the most important because of the clinical significance of HIT (38). HIT is seen in approximately 1% of patients receiving unfractionated heparin and generally appears five to seven days after therapy is begun or following exposure, such as during cardiopulmonary bypass. Although HIT is more common in surgical patients and those receiving intravenous heparin, it is dosage-independent and may even occur with low-dose heparin prophylaxis. Thrombocytopenia is a consequence of platelet activation and aggregation following heparin-platelet factor 4-IgG immune complex deposition. HIT is often complicated by severe venous or arterial thrombosis.

HIT patients may present with arterial thrombotic events such as myocardial infarction, stroke or limb ischemia, or venous thromboembolic disease such as deep venous thrombosis or pulmonary embolism as a consequence of platelet and coagulation activation. Heparin must be stopped immediately when HIT is suspected by recent thrombocytopenia onset or a decrease in the platelet count of 30–50%. The diagnosis should be confirmed by the determination of antibodies to platelet factor 4 in serum.

The most readily available test for HIT is an enzyme immunoassay that detects IgG, IgM, and IgA antibodies. Recent publications have shown that IgG is the most pathogenic, and that its concentration correlates with the risk of thrombosis (39,40). A positive immunoassay is nearly 100% sensitive for HIT but only 60% specific. The *serotonin release assay* determines the clinical significance of the antibodies and is helpful in some patients. Because of the risk of thrombosis, alternative anticoagulants such as the direct thrombin inhibitors argatroban or lepirudin must be initiated. Since patients do not tend to bleed, platelet transfusion is not necessary and may aggravate the thrombotic complications.

Non-Immune-Mediated Thrombocytopenia

Disseminated intravascular coagulation (DIC) is uncontrolled activation of coagulation with massive production of thrombin, causing coagulation factor deficiencies and platelet consumption. Acute DIC is seen in critically ill patients with bacterial sepsis, viral infections, acute intoxications, trauma, or obstetric complications, and in rare malignancies such as acute promyelocytic leukemia (M3) and some adenocarcinomas. The diagnosis of DIC requires a clinical history of an inciting event, D-dimer levels 50–100× normal, thrombocytopenia, microangiopathic hemolytic anemia with schistocytes (MAHA), and prolonged clotting assays. Extreme D-dimer elevation alone is pathognomic, and other laboratory results may be bypassed.

In adults, *thrombotic thrombocytopenic purpura* (TTP) and *hemolytic-uremic syndrome* (HUS) are overlapping syndromes that include MAHA, thrombocytopenia, and end-organ damage from platelet thrombin (41). Although classic TTP was described as a pentad of thrombocytopenia, hemolytic anemia, fever, and neurological and renal abnormalities, few patients exhibit all five findings. Schistocytes in the peripheral blood film examination and thrombocytopenia are essential for the diagnosis of TTP-HUS, provided there is no alternative explanation. Most cases of TTP-HUS are sporadic, although a familial form exists. TTP-HUS also occurs in pregnancy, bone marrow transplant, or as a result of drugs such as ticlopidine. Many patients with TTP have an autoantibody-mediated acquired deficiency of von Willebrand factor (VWF)-cleaving protease, also known as ADAMTS13, resulting in the plasma accumulation of ultra-large VWF (ULVWF) multimers. These trigger spontaneous platelet aggregation (41,42,43).

HUS is characterized by thrombocytopenia, MAHA, and renal failure. Classic HUS occurs in children infected with *Escherichia coli* serotype O157:H7 from undercooked contaminated meat (44,45). Childhood HUS presents with hemorrhagic colitis, followed in a few days by MAHA. Although the platelet aggregation mechanism is not well understood, an *E. coli* verotoxin is thought to be implicated.

One laboratory feature that distinguishes TTP and HUS may be the plasma level of VWF-cleaving protease. Enzyme activity below 5% is specific for TTP, while it is expected to be normal in HUS (44). However, there is considerable overlap and the current understanding suggests that deficiency of VWF-cleaving protease alone is not sufficient to cause or diagnose TTP. Consequently, adults with HUS receive therapeutic plasma exchange like those with TTP.

Thrombocytosis

Thrombocytosis is defined as a platelet count $\geq 500,000/\mu L$, and is most commonly reactive to hemorrhage, hemolysis, infection, inflammation, asplenia, cancer, or iron deficiency. Patients with secondary thrombocytosis have few platelet-related symptoms (46).

Primary thrombocytosis is often $>1,000,000/\mu L$ and is caused by myeloproliferative disorders (MPD). Patients with polycythemia vera (PV) and essential thrombocythemia (ET) are at significant risk of arterial and, less commonly, venous thromboembolic events due to high counts and functionally abnormal platelets. The microscopic review of the peripheral smear shows normal platelet morphology in reactive thrombocytosis but a variety of aberrant forms in MPDs. Microvascular ischemia of the digits or central nervous system occurs spontaneously or during situational hypercoagulability, such as surgery, immobilization, and pregnancy in primary thrombocytosis. Additional risk factors for thrombosis include age >60 years, history of prior thrombosis, cardiovascular comorbidities and, for PV, erythrocytosis (47,48).

"Rebound" thrombocytosis after splenectomy can lead to thrombosis in patients with chronic idiopathic myelofibrosis (IMF, myelofibrosis with myeloid metaplasia, MMM). Although the thrombotic risk in patients with MPD is not directly related to platelet count, most events occur when it is >600,000/μL.

Mucocutaneous bleeding is less common than thrombosis. Paradoxically, bleeding occurs with platelet counts >1,500,000/μL in about 12% and 23% of patients with ET and PV, respectively. Bleeding also occurs in the setting of acquired von Willebrand disease.

Flow Cytometry (FCM)

FCM is a rapid automated technique for establishing the immunophenotype of hematopoietic neoplasms (49). Fresh saline suspensions of blood or bone marrow neoplastic cells are stained with fluorochrome-tagged monoclonal antibodies and passed single-file through a capillary tube illuminated by single or double laser sources at 488 and 635 ηm (49). Photodetectors convert light to voltage and generate four to six simultaneous antibody color combination analyses of the target cell populations.

Indications for FCM

- Diagnosis and classification of lymphomas, leukemias, and other hematologic malignancies by detection and immunophenotyping of clonal cell populations including κ and λ light chain restriction (50)
- Detection of aberrant cell populations such as T LYMPHs that co-express B or NK markers
- Detection of immunodeficiency syndromes through T or B LYMPH subset quantitation

- Detection of immature cells and blasts; T or B LYMPH precursors, NK cell precursors, myelocytic cells, myeloblasts, or monocytic precursors
- Therapy monitoring by assessment of residual lymphoma or leukemia cells called minimal residual disease (MRD)
- Establishment of therapeutic targets with monoclonal antibodies specific to cell surface antigens such as CD20, CD30, CD33, and CD52
- Assessment of prognostic markers such as CD38 and ZAP-70 for CLL
- Determination of leukocyte adhesion molecules, cytoplasmic enzymes, and markers

Sample Requirements for FCM

- Cell viability >70% is necessary for analysis. However, limited analysis is possible on low viability samples by using markers such as 7AAD and selectively gating on viable cells
- At least 800,000 to 1 million cells are needed for complete lymphoma or leukemia immunophenotype analysis
- Cellular yield and viability are better with blood, bone marrow, and body fluids than with soft tissue such as lymph nodes
- For soft tissue, fresh unfixed tissue fragments are essential for preparing cell suspensions
- Gentle tissue disaggregation is recommended for optimal cell yield and viability
- Cells and tissues preserved in Hanks balanced salt solution or RPMI 1640 are viable for analysis for 4 days

Table 38. Specimens for FCM

Markers	Specimen	Additive	Storage
CD3/CD4, CD4, CD4/CD8	Blood	Dry K$_2$EDTA (lavender closure)	23–28 °C
		Dry Li or Na heparin (green closure)	
		Liquid sodium heparin syringe	
Other cell markers	Body fluid	Dry K$_2$EDTA, dry Li or Na heparin, Hanks or RPMI	4–8 °C
	Bone marrow	Hanks balanced salt solution or RPMI	
	Tissue	Hanks balanced salt solution or RPMI	

FCM Analysis Sequence

1. Disaggregate tissue and prepare mononuclear cell suspension.
2. Perform cytospin smear review of cell suspension.
3. Test for total yield and cell viability.
4. Select antibody and fluorochrome combinations from disease panels.
5. Stain cells for three or four-color staining analysis.
6. Introduce sample to flow cytometer, which may have multiple lasers and detectors.
7. Analyze results.

Analysis of FCM Results

Light Scatter Analysis: Side- (SSC) and Forward-Scatter (FSC) Signals (51)

- Forward scatter intensity is proportional to *cell volume.*
- Side scatter intensity is proportional to *surface complexity and cytoplasmic granularity.*
- Side scatter is also used to detect surface and cytoplasmic immunophenotyping dyes.

Scatterplot Analysis

- Flow artifacts such as cell clumping and nonspecific binding
- Intensity of fluorochrome expression: dim vs. bright signal
- Abnormal expression of normal antigens
- Aberrant marker co-expression; for example, CD5 (T marker) and CD20 (B marker) in CLL/SLL; low CD45 in immature cells
- Cross-lineage antigen expression such as myeloid markers on lymphoid cells or lymphoid markers on myeloid cells
- Relative percentages of neoplastic cells
- Loss of normal antigens; for example, loss of CD5 or CD7 in T-cell proliferative conditions; loss of CD13 or CD33 in some myeloid leukemias
- Selective gating; mononuclear, lymphoid, monocyte, blast, and granulocyte gates

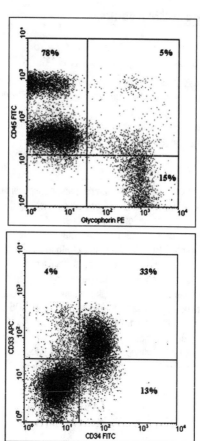

Figure 17. FCM scatterplots.
- Top: Comparison of glycophorin and CD45
- Bottom: Comparison of CD34 and CD33

FCM Differential and Manual Blast Counts

- FCM is excellent for cell *lineage* identification (51).
- FCM analyzes the *mononuclear* cell population, which excludes PMNs, SEGs, BANDs, EOS, and BASOs.
- Blast counts are relative, based on sample preparation, concentration method by Ficoll separation, and gating strategies. Therefore, FCM cannot be used alone for estimating and reporting blast counts.
- Because FCM is an *independent measurement*, results have to be correlated with specimen morphology, cell counts, and histologic findings.

Table 39. Cell Lineages by FCM

	Markers
B-cells	CD45, tDt, CD34, CD10, CD38, CD19, CD79, CD20, CD22, HLA-DR, IgD, IgM, κ, λ
T-cells	CD45, CD34, tDt, CD2, CD3, cCD3, CD5, CD7, CD4/CD8, TCR
Myeloid	CD45, CD34, CD117, CD13, CD33, CD64, CD15, CD65, CD11b, CD16, CD35, CD14, CD10
Monocytic	CD45, CD34, CD13, CD33, CD64, HLA-DR, CD64, CD15, CD11b, CD36, CD4, CD14, CD16
Erythroid	CD45 (variable), CD71, CD36, CD235, glycophorin-A
Meg	CD31, CD41, CD61, CD62, factor VIIIag
NK cells	CD2, cCD3, CD56, CD57
γ/δ	TCR/γ/δ, CD2, CD3, CD4/CD8 neg

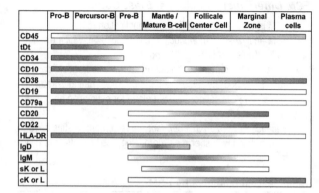

Figure 18. B-LYMPH FCM maturation and differentiation markers (51).
sκ or λ, surface κ or λ; cκ or λ, cytoplasmic κ or λ.

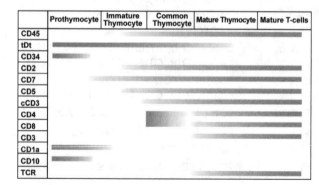

Figure 19. T-LYMPH FCM maturation and differentiation markers (52).
cCD3, cytoplasmic CD3; CD1a and CD10 are expressed in acute T-cell
leukemias.

	Blast	Promyelocyte	Myelocyte	Metamyelocyte	Band	Neutrophil
CD45						
tDt						
CD34						
CD117						
CD13						
CD33						
CD64						
CD15						
CD11b						
CD16						
CD65						
CD35						
CD14						
CD10						

Figure 20. Myeloid FCM maturation and differentiation markers (53).

	Monoblast	Promonocytes	Monocytes
CD45			
CD34			
CD13			
CD33			
HLA-DR			
CD64			
CD15			
CD11b			
CD36			
CD4			
CD14			
CD16			

Figure 21. Monocytic FCM maturation and differentiation markers.

Cytochemical and Special Histochemical Stains

Enzyme cytochemical stains are useful for rapid diagnosis of myeloid vs. monocytic leukemias. However, these have mostly been replaced by flow cytometry cell marker studies (54).

Histochemical stains relevant to hematology include the Prussian blue iron stain for hemosiderin pigment and the trichrome and reticulin stains for demonstrating bone marrow fibrosis.

Table 40. Cytochemical and Histochemical Stains

Stain	Detects
Myeloperoxidase (MPO)	
Sudan black B (SBB)	Blast to mature stages of the
Naphthol AS-D chloroacetate "specific" esterase	myeloid lineage
Nonspecific esterase (NSE)	Early to mature stages of the monocytic lineage
Periodic acid Schiff (PAS)	Cytoplasmic glycogen in erythroblasts in erythroleukemia and in some lymphoblasts in ALL
Tartrate-resistant acid phosphatase (TRAP)	Hairy cells in hairy cell leukemia
Neutrophil (leukocyte) alkaline phosphatase (NAP, LAP)	Differentiates CML from PV and leukemoid reaction
Reticulin	Detection of early collagen (reticulin) fibers in bone marrow fibrosis, called myelofibrosis
Iron (hemosiderin)	Hemosiderin pigment in macrophages and in erythroid precursors such as ringed sideroblasts
Congo red	Amyloid deposits

Immunohistochemical Stains (IPOX)

Limited immunophenotyping for cell marker analysis is possible on bone marrow or lymph node smears and formalin fixed tissue sections. Cellular antigen epitopes are altered during formalin fixation, thus requiring that an antigen retrieval technique is applied to the smears and tissue sections before incubating with antibodies. Immunohistochemical stains are used to visualize immuno-architecture and localize rare abnormal cells, viruses, and bacteria.

Table 41. IPOX Stains on Fixed Tissues

Cell Type	Marker
B-LYMPH	CD20, CD79a, κ or λ
T-LYMPH	CD2, CD3, CD4, CD5, CD7, CD8
NK cell	CD56, CD57
Plasma cell	CD138 and CD79a; κ or λ
Myeloid	CD15, CD117, and (MPO)
Monocytic	CD14, CD68
Hodgkin lymphoma	CD15, CD30, PAX-5

Cytogenetics, Fluorescent In Situ Hybridization (FISH), and PCR

Molecular diagnostic techniques are used increasingly in hematopathology for diagnosis, molecular classification, prognosis, and minimal residual disease detection. The 2001 WHO classification of the hematolymphoid tumors is based on *cytogenetic and molecular* findings in addition to time-honored morphology and immunophenotype.

Cytogenetics (Karyotyping)

Cytogenetics techniques employ Giemsa or Wright stains, or stain modifications, to microscopically evaluate the *banding patterns of metaphase chromosomes* from cultured LYMPHs or blasts. Specimens include blood, bone marrow, amniotic fluid, and tissues, which must be delivered to the laboratory immediately after collection to preserve cell viability. Tissue samples must be transported and stored at 4 °C to avoid proteolytic digestion. Sterility of the specimen prior to and during culture is essential to yield meaningful results; bacteria and fungal contamination outgrow the cells of interest (55).

In the laboratory, blood and bone marrow are cultured in suspension, while amniotic fluid, chorionic villi, and solid tissue are grown in a monolayer fixed to a tissue culture surface. Cells from lymph nodes are first disaggregated with collagenase and then placed on culture medium. Bone marrow cells typically require 24–48 hours to grow, while LYMPHs must be stimulated with a mitogen such as phyto-hemagglutinin, and require 72–96 hours.

After reaching maximum growth, cells are harvested, adhered to glass slides and stained for chromosome analysis. A trained microscopist counts the chromosomes in each cell and evaluates their morphology using 1000x light microscopy and computer-assisted imaging when available. To prevent artifactual errors, chromosomes of at least 15–20 abnormal cells are analyzed. Normal cells grow more rapidly than malignant cells in culture, so abnormal chromosomal morphology may be seen in only 1–5% of cells.

FISH

Dye-impregnated *molecular probes* are used in FISH to identify inter-phase genes, mutations, microdeletions, or chromosomal rearrange-ments. Cell culture is unnecessary; however, metaphase cells may also be stained. Probes are chosen to detect genetic findings of interest. FISH provides sensitivity at the *oligonucleotide* level, conventional cytogenetics at the *chromosome* level. To avoid error, the microscopist uses fluorescence microscopy to evaluate at least 20 cells because, as in cytogenetics, the abnormalities may be seen in only 1–5% of cells. However, FISH is more sensitive than cytogenetics in tumor cell suspensions and tissue sections.

Cytogenetics and FISH are employed to evaluate hematological disorders for clonal abnormalities. They help establish disease identity and provide prognostic information. Cytogenetics is used to classify leukemias as *therapy-related* or *de novo*, monitor *remission*, and confirm *stem cell transplant* engraftment. Further, both methods aid in determining which lineages are involved in MPDs.

Specific karyotype abnormalities have not been detected for most myeloid disorders, and abnormalities that are present may not always characterize the primary pathogenetic events. Currently, only chronic myelogenous leukemia (CML) has a specific chromosomal anomaly, the Philadelphia chromosome, t(9;22) (q34;q11.2) or a variant of this translocation (Table 42). Most hematologic diseases potentially undergo clonal evolution, and cytogenetic or molecular changes signal an accelerated stage or transformation to an acute process. Besides providing prognostic data, cytogenetics and FISH allow clearer understanding of the molecular biology of the disease. Ultimately, this information will be used to develop targeted therapy.

Polymerase Chain Reaction (PCR) and Reverse Transcription PCR (RT-PCR)

Polymerase chain reaction (PCR): PCR detects one genetically abnormal cell in 1000–20,000 normal cells from blood, fresh tissue, or fixed tissue (56).

Reverse transcription polymerase chain reaction (RT-PCR): Complementary DNA (cDNA) from viral or other mRNA is used for analysis of genomic abnormalities. RT-PCR sensitivity is 1 in 200,000 cells. RT-PCR is well suited for minimal disease detection in CML or ALL.

False positive PCR results in nonmalignant conditions have been reported, so the diagnosis of malignancy should be based on the combination of morphology, immunophenotypic data, molecular diagnostics, and clinical condition of the patient. False negative PCR, RT-PCR, and FISH may result from sampling problems or poor tissue preservation.

Table 42. Cytogenetic Abnormalities in Hematologic Malignancies

Myeloproliferative Disorders (MPDs)

Diagnosis	Abnormal genes or chromosomes
Chronic myelogenous leukemia, chronic phase (CML)	t(9;22)(q34.1;q11.2); BCR/ABL
CML, accelerated or blast phase	+8; i(17q); +19; +Ph'
Polycythemia vera (PV)	+8; −7; del(7q); del(11q); del(13q); del(20q)
Chronic idiopathic myelofibrosis with myeloid metaplasia (MMM)	+8; −7; del(7q); del(11q); del(13q); del(20q)
Essential thrombocythemia (ET)	+8; del(13q)

Myelodysplastic Syndromes (MDSs)

Diagnosis	Abnormal genes or chromosomes
Myelodysplastic syndrome with isolated del(5q)	del(5)(q13q33); del(5)(q22q33)
Chronic myelomonocytic leukemia (CMML)	−7; del(7q); +8; abnormalities of 12p
Refractory anemia (RA); RA with ringed sideroblasts (RARS); RA with excess blasts (RAEB)	−5; del(5q); −7; del(7q); +8; del(20q)

Acute Myeloblastic Leukemia (AML) with Recurrent Cytogenetic Abnormalities

WHO name	FAB name	Abnormal genes or chromosomes
AML with t(8;21)	M2	t(8;21)(q22;q22); *AML1; ETO*
AML with inv or t16	M4Eo	inv(16)(p12;q22); t(16;16)(p13;q22); *CBFβ; MYH11*
Acute promyelocytic leukemia	M3	t(15;17)(q22;q12); *PML; RARα*
AML with 11q23 (MLL) abnormalities	M5	t(9;11)(p21;q23); t(11;19)(q23;p13.1); t(11;19)(q23;p13.3); *AF9; MLL; ENL*
AML with multilineage dysplasia	M1, M6	−5; del(5q); −7; del(7q); +8; del(11q); del(20q); +21; translocations involving 3q21 and 3q26; t(9;22)(q34.1;q11.2)

Mature Lymphoid Neoplasms

Lymphoid neoplasm	Abnormal genes or chromosomes
Chronic lymphocytic leukemia (CLL), small lymphocytic lymphoma (SLL)	+12; del(13q); del(11q23–24); 14q+; del(17p13)
Lymphoplasmacytic lymphoma, Waldenström macroglobulinemia	t(9;14)(p13;q32); *PAX5; IGH*
Plasma cell myeloma	t(11;14)(q13;q32); *CCND1; BCL1*
Marginal zone B-cell lymphoma (MALT)	+3; t(11;18)(q21;q21)
Follicular lymphoma	t(14;18)(q32;q21); t(18;22)(q21;q11.2); +7; +18 del(6q); del/t(3)(q27); IGH; BCL2; IGL

Continued

Table 42. (continued)

Mature Lymphoid Neoplasms (continued)

Lymphoid neoplasm	Abnormal genes or chromosomes
Mantle cell lymphoma	t(11;14)(q13;32); CCND1; BCL1
Burkitt lymphoma	t(8;14)(q24;q32), MYC, IGH; t(2;8)(p12;q24), IGK, MYC; t(8;22)(q24;q11.2), MYC, IGL
T-cell anaplastic large cell lymphoma (80–90%)	t(2;5)/NPM-ALK and variant ALK translocations
Extranodal marginal zone lymphomas (20–30%)	t(11;18)/API2-MALT1; t(14;18)/MALT1-IgH

Precursor B-Lymphoblastic Leukemia and Lymphoma: ALL L1 and L2

t(1;19)(q23;p13.3); PBX; E2A
t(9;22)(q34;q11.2); ABL; BCR
t(11;19)(q23;p13); MLL; ENL
t(12;21)(p13q22); TEL; AML
Hyperdiploidy (modal number 50–56)
11q23 rearrangements, including:
- t(1;11)(p32;q23); AF1P; MLL
- t(4;11)(q21;q23); AF4; MLL

Precursor T-Lymphoblastic Leukemia and Lymphoma: ALL L1 and L2

Rearrangements at 14q11.2; 7q35; 7p14–15; T-cell receptor loci; del(9p); CDKN2A; translocations at 1p32; TAL1

del, deletion; inv, inversion; i, isochromosome; r, ring; t, translocation

Table 43. Chromosome Breakage Syndromes in Hematologic Malignancies

Type of Malignancy or Disorder	Clinical Features
Fanconi anemia with increased risk of AML and progressive bone marrow failure	Pancytopenia, pre- or postnatal growth retardation, hypoplastic or missing thumbs, possible arm deformation, brownish pigmentation of skin
Ataxia telangiectasia with various leukemias and solid tumors	Ataxia with degeneration of central nervous system, telangiectasia on face, deficiency in cellular immunity, degenerative, growth retardation

Table 44. Genetic Abnormalities in Pediatric B-Lineage ALL

Favorable Prognosis	Unfavorable Prognosis
Hyperdiploidy (>52 chromosomes)	t(1;19)/E2A-PBX1
t(12;21)/TEL-AML1	t(9;22)/BCR-ABL1
	11q23/MLL gene rearrangements
	Hypodiploidy (<40 chromosomes)

Table 45. Genetic Abnormalities and Related Hematologic Malignancies (55)

Genetic Abnormality	Hematologic Malignancy	Molecular Pathogenesis	Detection
t(9;22)/BCR-ABL1	Chronic myeloid leukemia (CML, 100%) Ph+ adult acute lymphoblastic leukemia (~20%) Ph+ pediatric acute lymphoblastic leukemia (3%)	Chimeric fusion protein with deregulation of ABL tyrosine kinase	RT-PCR > FISH
del 4q12/FIP1L1-PDGFRA	Hypereosinophilic syndrome/ chronic eosinophilic leukemia (subset of cases) (54)	Deregulation of PDGFRα receptor tyrosine kinase	FISH > RT-PCR
t(15;17)/PML-RARα	Acute promyelocytic leukemia (APL, 100%)	Chimeric fusion protein; interference with myeloid maturation and differentiation	RT-PCR > FISH
t(8;21)/AML1-ETO, inv(16) or t(16;16)/ CBFB-MYH11	Acute myeloblastic leukemia (AML, 10%) Acute myelomonocytic leukemia with abnormal eosinophils (AMML-Eo)	Chimeric fusion protein affecting the core binding factor (CBF) transcriptional regulatory pathway; aberrant effects on myeloid cell proliferation and differentiation	RT-PCR; FISH
c-kit (D816V)	Mast cell disease	Activation of tyrosine kinase	PCR

112

FLT3 mutations	AML (20–30%)	Point mutation resulting in constitutive activity of FLT3 tyrosine kinase and cell proliferation	DNA PCR
JAK2 mutation	Chronic MPDs excluding CML: P vera(~90%), chronic idiopathic myelofibrosis, essential thrombocytosis (~50%); rarely seen in myelodysplastic syndrome or atypical MDS/MDP	Single G>T point mutation producing V617F amino acid substitution; results in loss of feedback control and constitutive activation of Jak2 tyrosine kinase	DNA PCR
t(12;21)/TEL-AML1	Childhood B-precursor acute lymphoblastic leukemia (20%)	Chimeric fusion protein; disruption of CBF transcriptional regulatory pathway; abnormal effects on Tel transcriptional function	RT-PCR; FISH
t(1;19)/E2A-PBX1	Childhood pre-B cell ALL (3%)	Chimeric fusion protein; interference with normal early B-cell development	RT-PCR

113

Continued

Table 45. (continued)

Genetic Abnormality	Hematologic Malignancy	Molecular Pathogenesis	Detection
11q 23/MLL translocations	Childhood (mainly infant) B-lineage ALL (5%)	Chimeric fusion proteins; disruption of MLL-mediated regulation of hematopoiesis	FISH; RT-PCR
	Adult de novo AML, usually monocytic (rare)		
	Subset of secondary AML (after DNA topoisomerase II agent exposure)		
t(11;14)/BCL1-IgH	Mantle cell lymphoma/leukemia (100%)	Over expression of cyclin-D1/Bcl-1	FISH >> PCR
t(14;18)BCL2-IgH	Follicular lymphoma (80–90%)	Over expression of Bcl-2 protein	FISH > PCR
	Diffuse large cell lymphoma (20–30%)		
t(8;14)/and variant c-myc translocation	Burkitt lymphoma (100%)	Over expression of c-myc	FISH
t(11;18)/API2-MALT1 t(14;18)MALT1-IgH	Marginal zone lymphoma (20–30%)	Upregulation of NF-κB transduction pathway	FISH, PT-PCR
(2;5)/NPM-ALK	Anaplastic large cell lymphoma (ALCL), 80–90%	Activation of ALK-tyrosine kinase	FISH, RT-PCR for NPM-ALK mRNA

References

1. CLSI Document H3-A5, Vol 23 No 32. Procedures for the collection of diagnostic blood specimens by venipuncture; approved standard, 5th ed. Wayne, PA: Clinical and Laboratory Standards Institute, 2003.

2. CLSI Document H4-A4, Vol. 19 No 16. Procedures and devices for the collection of diagnostic blood specimens by skin puncture; approved standard, 4th ed. Wayne, PA: Clinical and Laboratory Standards Institute, 1999.

3. McCall RE, Tankersley CM. Phlebotomy essentials, 2nd ed. Philadelphia: Lippincott, 1998.

4. Hippel T, Clark K. Routine testing in hematology. In: Rodak BF, Fritsma GA, Doig K, eds. Hematology clinical principles and applications, 3rd ed. Philadelphia: Elsevier, 2007.

5. Craig FE. Flow cytometry. In: McKenzie SB. Clinical laboratory hematology. Upper Saddle River, NJ: Prentice Hall, 2003.

6. Becton-Dickinson Vacutainer. http://www.bd.com/vacutainer/ (Accessed November 2006).

7. Perkins SL. Normal blood and bone marrow values in humans. In: Greer JP, Foerster J, Lukens JN, et al., eds. Wintrobe's clinical hematology, 11th ed. Philadelphia: Lippincott, Williams and Wilkins, 2004.

8. Miers MK, Longanbach SA, Chapman DH. Automated cell counting instrumentation and point of care testing. In: Rodak BF, Fritsma GA, Doig K, eds. Hematology clinical principles and applications, 3rd ed. Philadelphia: Elsevier, 2007.

9. Maedel LB, Doig K. Examination of the peripheral blood smear and correlation with the complete blood count. In: Rodak BF, Fritsma GA, Doig K, eds. Hematology clinical principles and applications, 3rd ed. Philadelphia: Elsevier, 2007.

10. Hirscher H. [In memoriam of Dr. Joseph Arneth.] Munch Med Wochenschr 1956;98:1251–2.

11. LeClair SJ. Morphologic and distributive leukocyte disorders. In: Rodak BF, Fritsma GA, Doig K, eds. Hematology clinical principles and applications, 3rd ed. Philadelphia: Elsevier, 2007.

12. Krause JR. Bone marrow overview. In: Rodak BF, Fritsma GA, Doig K, eds. Hematology clinical principles and applications, 3rd ed. Philadelphia: Elsevier, 2007.

13. Vajpaee N, Graham SS, Bem S. Basic examination of blood and bone marrow. In: McPherson RA, Pincus MR, eds. Henry's clinical diagnosis and management by laboratory methods, 21st ed. Philadelphia: Saunders-Elsevier, 2006.

14. Kremer M, Quintanilla ML, Nahrig J, et al. Immunohistochemistry in bone marrow pathology: a useful adjunct for morphologic diagnosis. Virchows Arch 2005;447:920–37.

15. Elghetany TM, Banki K. Erythrocytic disorders. In: McPherson RA, Pincus MR, eds. Henry's clinical diagnosis and management by laboratory methods, 21st ed. Philadelphia: Saunders-Elsevier, 2006.

16. Dallalio G, Law E, Means RT Jr. Hepcidin inhibits in vitro erythroid colony formation at reduced erythropoietin concentration. Blood 2006;107:2702–4.

17. Camaschella C. Understanding iron hemostasis through genetic analysis of hemochromatosis and related disorders. Blood 2005;106:3710–7.

18. Centers for Disease Control and Prevention. Publication 77-82666. Atlanta: CDC, 1976.

19. Rosse WF, Hillmen P, Schreiber AD. Immune-mediated hemolytic anemia. Hematology 2004: Am Soc Hematol Educ Program Book 2004;48–62.

20. Reardon JE, Marques MB. Laboratory evaluation and transfusion support of patients with autoimmune hemolytic anemia. Am J Clin Pathol. 2006;125 Suppl:S71–7.

21. Garraty G. Drug-induced immune hemolytic anemia—the last decade [review]. Immunohematol 2004;20(3):138–46.

22. Vardiman JW, Brunning RD, Harris NL. Chronic myeloproliferative diseases. In: Jaffe ES, Harris NL, Stein H, Vardiman JW, eds. Pathology and genetics of tumors of hematopoietic and lymphoid tissues. Lyon: IARC Press, 2001.

23. Goldman JM. Myeloproliferative and myelodysplastic syndromes: the future. Hematol Oncol Clin North Am 2003;17:1261–9.

24. Brunning RD, Head D, Bennett JM. Myelodysplastic syndromes. In: Jaffe ES, Harris NL, Stein H, Vardiman JW, eds. Pathology and genetics of tumors of hematopoietic and lymphoid tissues. Lyon: IARC Press, 2001.

25. Steensma DP, Bennett JM. The myelodysplastic syndromes: diagnosis and treatment. Mayo Clin Proc 2006;81:104–30.

26. Catenacci DV, Schiller GJ. Myelodysplastic syndromes: a comprehensive review. Blood Rev 2005;19:301–19.

27. Greenberg P, Cox C, LeBeau M, et al. International scoring system for evaluating prognosis in myelodysplastic syndromes. Blood 1997;89:2079–88.

28. Brunning RD, Bennett JM, Vardiman JW. Acute myeloid leukemia. In: Jaffe ES, Harris NL, Stein H, Vardiman JW, eds. Pathology and genetics of tumors of hematopoietic and lymphoid tissues. Lyon: IARC Press, 2001.

29. Lichtman MA, Segel GB. Uncommon phenotypes of acute myelogenous leukemia: basophilic, mast cell, eosinophilic, and myeloid dendritic cell subtypes: a review. Blood Cells Mol Dis 2005;35:370–83.

30. Slack GW, Wizniak J, Dabbagh L, et al. Flow cytometric detection of ZAP-70 in chronic lymphocytic leukemia: correlation with immunocytochemistry and western blot analysis. Arch Pathol Lab Med 2007;131:50–6.

31. Cohen AM, Cycowitz Z, Mittelman M, et al. The incidence of pseudothrombocytopenia in automatic blood analyzers. Haematologia (Budap) 2000;30:117–21.

32. Girard DE, Kumar KL, McAfee JH. Hematologic effects of acute alcohol abuse. Hematol Oncol Clin North Am 1987;1:321–34.

33. Peck-Radosavljevic M. Thrombocytopenia in liver disease. Can J Gastroenterol 2000;14 Suppl D:60D–66D.

34. Zucker-Franklin D, Cao Y. Megakaryocytes of human immunodeficiency virus-infected individuals express viral RNA. Proc Natl Acad Sci USA 1989;86:5595–9.

35. Miguez-Burbano MJ, Jackson J Jr, Hadrigan S. Thrombocytopenia in HIV disease: clinical relevance, physiopathology, and management. Curr Med Chem Cardiovasc Hematol Agents 2005;3:365–76.

36. Balduini CL, Iolascon A, Savoia A. Inherited thrombocytopenias: from genes to therapy. Haematologica 2002;87:860–80.

37. Kuwana M, Okazaki Y, Satoh T, et al. Initial laboratory findings useful for predicting the diagnosis of idiopathic thrombocytopenic purpura. Am J Med 2005;118:1026–33.

38. Warkentin TE, Greinacher A. Heparin-induced thrombocytopenia: recognition, treatment, and prevention: the seventh ACCP conference on antithrombotic and thrombolytic therapy. Chest 2004;126:311S–37S.

39. Warkentin TE, Sheppard JA, Moore JC, et al. Laboratory testing for the antibodies that cause heparin-induced thrombocytopenia: how much class do we need? J Lab Clin Med 2005;146:341–6.

40. Zwicker JI, Uhl L, Huang WY, et al. Thrombosis and ELISA optical density values in hospitalized patients with heparin-induced thrombocytopenia. J Thromb Haemost 2004;2:2133–7.

41. Sadler JE, Moake JL, Myata T, George JN. Recent advances in thrombotic thrombocytopenic purpura. Hematology (Am Soc Hematol Educ Program) 2004;407–23.

42. George JN. The role of ADAMTS13 in the pathogenesis of thrombotic thrombocytopenic purpura-hemolytic uremic syndrome. Clin Adv Hematol Oncol 2005;3:627–32.

43. Furlan M, Robles R, Galbusera M, et al. von Willebrand factor-cleaving protease in thrombotic thrombocytopenic purpura and the hemolytic-uremic syndrome. N Engl J Med 1998;339:1578–84.

44. Tsai H-M, Lian EC-Y. Antibodies to von Willebrand factor-cleaving protease in acute thrombotic thrombocytopenic purpura. N Engl J Med 1998;339:1585–94.

45. Blackall DP, Marques MB. Hemolytic uremic syndrome revisited: Shiga toxin, factor H, and fibrin generation. Am J Clin Pathol 2004;121:S81–8.

46. El-Moneim AA, Kratz CP, Boll S, et al. Essential versus reactive thrombocythemia in children: retrospective analyses of 12 cases. Pediatr Blood Cancer 2006 Dec 14; [Epub ahead of print].

47. Finazzi G, Rambaldi A, Guerini V, et al. Risk of thrombosis in patients with essential thrombocythemia and polycythemia vera according to JAK2 V617F mutation status. Haematologica 2007;92:135–6.

48. Griesshammer M. Risk factors for thrombosis and bleeding and their influence on therapeutic decisions in patients with essential thrombocythemia. Semin Thromb Hemost 2006;32(4 Pt 2):372–80.

49. Szczepanski T, van der Velden VH, van Dongen JJ. Flow-cytometric immunophenotyping of normal and malignant lymphocytes. Clin Chem Lab Med 2006;44:775–96.

50. Del Vecchio L, Brando B, Lanza F, et al. Recommended reporting format for flow cytometry diagnosis of acute leukemia. Haematologica 2004;89:594–8.

51. Chen W, Karandikar NJ, McKenna RW, Kroft SH. Stability of leukemia-associated immunophenotypes in precursor B-lymphoblastic leukemia/lymphoma: a single institution experience. Am J Clin Pathol 2007;127:39–46.

52. Wood BL, Borowitz MJ. The flow cytometric evaluation of hematopoietic neoplasm. In: McPherson RA, Pincus MR, eds. Henry's clinical diagnosis and management by laboratory methods, 21st ed. Philadelphia: Saunders-Elsevier, 2006.

53. Viswanatha DS, Larson RS. Molecular diagnosis of hematopoietic neoplasms; the flow cytometric evaluation of hematopoietic neoplasm. In: McPherson RA, Pincus MR, eds. Henry's clinical diagnosis and management by laboratory methods, 21st ed. Philadelphia: Saunders-Elsevier, 2006.

54. Reddy VVB. Selected case studies in hematopathology: application of current ancillary techniques in diagnosis. Adv Exp Med Biol 2005;563:112–24.

55. Hilliard NJ, Warraich I, Kruspe R, et al. Idiopathic eosinophilia associated CMML-2 with over expression of the ETV6 gene. Lab Medicine 2007;38;100–2.

56. Stein CK. Applications of cytogenetics in modern pathology In: McPherson RA, Pincus MR, eds. Henry's clinical diagnosis and management by laboratory methods, 21st ed. Philadelphia: Saunders-Elsevier, 2006:1260.

INDEX